Caregiver Renewed:

Developing an Inquisitive Mind for Medical Issues

by

Minori Yoshioka
Gerald R. Gordon
Susumu Kondo

Asahi Press

音声再生アプリ「リスニング・トレーナー」を使った音声ダウンロード

朝日出版社開発のアプリ、「リスニング・トレーナー（リストレ）」を使えば、教科書の音声をスマホ、タブレットに簡単にダウンロードできます。どうぞご活用ください。

◉ アプリ【リスニング・トレーナー】の使い方

《アプリのダウンロード》

App Store または Google Play から「リスニング・トレーナー」のアプリ（無料）をダウンロード

App Storeはこちら▶

Google Playはこちら▶

《アプリの使い方》

① アプリを開き「コンテンツを追加」をタップ
② 画面上部に【15672】を入力しDoneをタップ

音声ストリーミング配信 》》》

この教科書の音声は、右記ウェブサイトにて無料で配信しています。

 https://text.asahipress.com/free/english/

Sources of Articles:
Medical News Today (Unit 1, 2, 4, 11, 12); *Chicago Tribune* (Unit 3); Reuters (Unit 5); WebMD (unit 7); Voice of America (Unit 6, 8, 13, 14, 15); *The Canberra Times* (Unit 9); Associated Press News (Unit 10)

Caregiver Renewed: Developing an Inquisitive Mind for Medical Issue
Copyright © 2021 by Asahi Press

Illustrations by Yuri Yoshioka
Photographs by iStockphoto

は し が き

　本テキストの執筆中、中国で新型コロナウイルスによる感染症が初めて確認され、瞬く間にウイルスが国境を越え、世界中で猛威を振るっていました。ウイルスの蔓延により、社会生活が急速に変化し、世界中の人々は、不安と恐怖、悲しみと孤独に苛まれました。WHOがこの感染症（COVID-19）をパンデミック（pandemic）と宣言しました。医療従事者の方々（caregivers: doctors, nurses, medical staff and anyone who works on the front lines）は寝食を忘れて命がけで治療の最前線で闘っておられました。ここに、自らを犠牲にして、思いやりと使命感を持って人々の命を助けてくれた勇者たちに、感謝の気持ちを述べたいと思います。そして、このコロナ禍が一刻も早く終息することを切に願っています。

　新型コロナウイルスとの闘いの中で、医療研究者たちは、ウイルスの感染経路、感染症状、ウイルスの特質の分析からワクチン開発まで、多岐にわたる研究成果を次々に公表し、情報は世界中で共有されています。今や医学専門書を開かずとも、インターネットやニュースアプリから簡単に様々な医療情報にアクセスできる時代となりましたが、この膨大な医療情報を十分に活用するために、読み手にはツールとしての、Medical Englishに対する読解力、つまり、医療及び健康問題に関するさまざまな英文記事に抵抗なく、文章構成、表現や語彙に慣れ親しんでいることが求められます。

　本テキストは、医療、薬学、看護、栄養や健康科学などの分野にフォーカスして作成し、題材は、Medical English Today, VOA News, AP News, Reuters, The Canberra Times などのインターネットソースから、世界で話題になっている医療と健康に関する記事を中心に選びました。テキストは、腰痛、がんの治療技術、電子タバコの危険性、恐怖症へのVR技術の応用、アスピリンの効能、ヒアルロン酸や食用昆虫など、身近で興味深い記事から構成される15のユニットに加えて、日常の使いやすい会話表現を紹介する "Useful Expressions" のセクションを設けています。また、各ユニットの終わりの "Coffee Break" では、記事のテーマについてより深い関心と理解が得られるように、関連するトピックや情報データを紹介しています。巻末には、人体の名称、病院の様々な診療科の英語表記、病名や難解な医学用語を解く鍵となる接辞リストを載せていますので、是非ご活用ください。

　最後に本書出版に惜しみないご尽力をくださった日比野忠氏と朝日出版社編集部の皆様に深く感謝の意を表します。

編著者一同

Contents

Unit 1

Vitamin D

⌘Pre-reading⌘

ビタミンDは骨格を健康な状態に保ち、免疫、内分泌や心血管系に対しても多くのプラス効果を発揮することがわかっています。ビタミンDは、私たちの健康維持にとって必要不可欠な栄養素ですが、それを過剰に摂取してしまうとどうなるのでしょうか。最新の研究によると、ビタミンDの過剰摂取は高齢者にリスクをもたらす事がわかってきました。

⌘Reading⌘

A new study on the effect of vitamin D found that too much may lead to slower reaction times and increase the risk of falling among older people. Vitamin D is an essential vitamin that helps build and maintain healthy bones and teeth. Without this, our bodies cannot absorb calcium, which is the main component of bone. Vitamin D may also protect 5 against cancer and diabetes. Our bodies synthesize vitamin D when sunlight reaches the skin. The amount of vitamin D that our skin produces depends on several factors, including where we live, season and skin pigmentation. During winter, vitamin D production may decrease or be completely absent. 10

We can also get vitamin D from salmon, sardines, canned tuna, oysters and shrimp. People who are vegetarians can obtain this vitamin by consuming egg yolks, mushrooms and fortified food products such as soy milk, cereal and oatmeal. It may be harder for some older adults to absorb vitamin D because they may not get regular sun exposure. In 15 this case, taking a vitamin supplement or a multivitamin that contains vitamin D may help boost bone health and improve memory. Studies have linked vitamin D deficiency to conditions such as dementia, depression, diabetes, autism, and schizophrenia.

While it is crucial to take vitamin D, excessive exposure can also pose 20 risks. A study led by scientists at Rutgers University found that older women who are overweight or obese who took more than three times the recommended daily dose of vitamin D had slower reaction times. They analyzed the effects of vitamin D on three groups of women aged 50-70 in a randomized controlled trial: 25

・The first group took the recommended daily dose of 600 IU.
・The second group took 2,000 IU.
・The third took 4,000 IU.

The results showed an improvement in memory and learning in the groups that took more than the recommended daily dose. However, the same groups also experienced a slowdown in reaction times. Scientists think that the slower reaction time may have negative outcomes such as potentially increasing the risk of falling and fractures. They believe that the team's findings indicate a slower reaction time may be the reason behind the increased risk of falls.

According to the scientists, taking 4,000 IU of vitamin D per day might not be a problem for young people, but it could lower older adults' ability to walk or catch their balance to avoid a fall. However, more studies are needed to determine whether slower reaction times are linked to an increase in the risk of falls and injuries.

🔊 Words & Phrases

[l. 8]　**pigmentation:** 色素沈着
[l. 13]　**fortified:** 強化された
[l. 18]　**dementia:** 痴呆症
[l. 19]　**autism:** 自閉症
[l. 19]　**schizophrenia:** 統合失調症
[l. 21]　**Rutgers University:** ラトガーズ大学 (1766 年創立、アメリカ合衆国ニュージャージー州にある州立総合研究大学)
[l. 25]　**randomized controlled trial:** ランダム化比較試験 (RCT)。ある試験的操作を行うこと以外は公平になるように、対象の集団を無作為に複数の群 (介入群 vs. 対照群、新治療を行う群 vs. 通常の治療のみの群など) に分け、その試験的操作の影響や効果を測定するための比較研究のこと。
[l. 26]　**IU:** International Units; 40 International Units = 1 microgram (mcg)

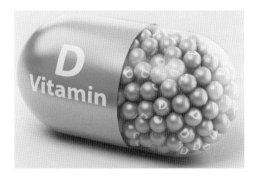

☑Vocabulary Check

Match each word in the box with the most appropriate definition shown below.

Words	Definitions	Words	Definitions
absorb		depression	
component		excessive	
diabetes		obese	
exposure		fracture	
deficiency		avoid	

Definitions:

a. a break or a crack in a bone, usually also involving injury to surrounding structures

b. the fact of experiencing something or being affected by it, or having no protection from something harmful

c. the state of feeling very unhappy and without hope for the future

d. very fat in a way that is dangerous for health

e. going beyond the usual, necessary, or proper limit or degree

f. a disease in which the body cannot control the level of sugar in the blood

g. a state of not having, or not having enough of, something that is needed

h. a part or element of a larger whole

i. take in and understand fully

j. keep away from or stop oneself from doing something

♀ Vocabulary Practice

Complete the following sentences with the words shown in the box. Change the grammatical form if necessary.

1. When I was a kid, I (   ) my leg by falling down the stairs.

2. He is (   ) because he eats too much fatty food and doesn't exercise.

3. Eating a balanced diet is one (   ) of having a healthy lifestyle.

4. Since my blood sugar levels are becoming so high, I'm worried about developing ( ).

5. You should ( ) too much sunlight or else you might get skin cancer.

6. A clear sign of ( ) is withdrawal from society and not wanting to leave the house.

7. Tom's ( ) drinking was becoming uncontrollable, and eventually he ended up going to a rehab center for help.

8. His doctor did a blood test on him to check if there were any signs of a vitamin ( ).

9. Some chemicals can be ( ) into our bodies through our skin.

10. Her ( ) to museums enriched her life because she learned about the history and culture of her country.

✍ Comprehension

Underline the words in each sentence that don't match the content of the article and correct them.

1. During winter, our bodies may produce more vitamin D because our skin doesn't get a lot of sunlight.
⇒ ( )

2. It may be harder for some older adults to absorb vitamin D because they take vitamin supplements.
⇒ ( )

3. Taking too much vitamin D can be good for you.
⇒ ( )

4. Slower reaction times always have negative outcomes, such as falling and memory loss.
⇒ ( )

5. According to the young people, taking 4,000 IU of vitamin D per day could lower older adults' ability to swim or drive a car.
⇒ ( )

ⓘ Coffee Break

What is vitamin D?

Despite the name, vitamin D is considered a pro-hormone and not actually a vitamin. Vitamins are nutrients that cannot be created by the body and therefore must be taken in through our diet. However, vitamin D can be synthesized by our body when sunlight hits our skin.

It is estimated that sensible sun exposure on bare skin for 5-10 minutes 2-3 times per week allows most people to produce sufficient vitamin D, but vitamin D breaks down quite quickly, meaning that stores can run low, especially in winter.

Source: https://www.myimyi.com/definition-of-vitamin-d/

📖 Words & Phrases

pro-hormone: プロホルモン
nutrient: 栄養素
synthesize: ～を合成する

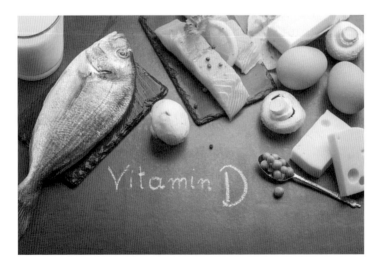

Unit 2

Dealing with Addiction

⌘Pre-reading⌘

この記事は薬物関連への依存障害について述べています。心理的症状及び身体的症状は、関連していてお互いに悪影響を及ぼし、依存者の生活の質、対人関係、社会への参加度を低下させる危険性があります。これらの兆候に気づくことにより依存障害の患者が必要な治療を受ける可能性が高まるのです。

⌘Reading⌘

What are the symptoms of addiction?

Addiction is a disease with a range of harmful conditions and behaviors. Recognizing these signs can help a person with addiction receive the treatment they need.

Doctors currently diagnose addictions under a category known as "substance-related and addictive disorders. 5

The main symptom of an addiction is a problematic pattern of use, which leads to clinically significant impairment or distress.

The specific symptoms vary according to the addictive disorder.

A person with a substance use disorder finds it difficult to control their 10 use of a specific substance. They continue using a substance or engaging in addictive behavior, even though they might be aware of the harm it can cause or when clear evidence of harm is apparent. Powerful cravings also characterize addiction. The individual may not be able to stop taking the addictive substance or doing the behavior despite expressing a desire to quit. 15

The signs and symptoms of substance use disorder can vary with the individual, the substance or behavior they are overusing, their family history, and their personal circumstances.

Overview

Substance use disorders have a range of psychological, physical, and social 20 effects that can drastically reduce people's quality of living.

While this article splits the symptoms into two categories, the reality is less clear. Many of these symptoms overlap and can lead to one another. An example of this overlap is when someone experiences the psychological effect of wanting to divert money from their regular food to purchase a substance, 25 and then not consuming enough nutrients. Likewise, relationship problems and a growing aversion to social interactions can lead to and worsen psychological problems, including depression and anxiety.

Psychological symptoms

10

Symptoms of addiction that cause mental disorders include the following. 30

- **An inability to stop using**: In many cases, such as a dependence on nicotine, alcohol, or other substances, a person will have made at least one serious but unsuccessful attempt to give up. This might also be physiological, as some substances, such as heroin, are chemically addictive and cause withdrawal symptoms if a person stops taking them. 35
- **Dealing with problems**: A person with addiction commonly feels the need to take the drug or carry out the behavior to deal with their problems.

Social symptoms

11

Substance use disorder can impact the way an individual socializes with 40 and relates to other people.

- **Sacrifices:** A person with substance dependence might give up some activities that previously brought them joy. For example, a person with alcohol use disorder may turn down an invitation to go camping or spend a day on a boat if no alcohol is available. 45
- **Dropping hobbies and activities:** As an addiction progresses, the individual may stop partaking in pastimes they enjoy. People who are dependent on tobacco, for example, might find they can no longer physically cope with taking part in their favorite sport.

⮂ Words & Phrases ───────────────────────

[l. 5] **substance-related and addictive disorders:** 物質関連障害。アルコールや薬物の乱用で生じる依存症

[l. 8] **clinically:** 臨床的に

[l. 8] **impairment:** 損傷、悪化

[l. 8] **distress:** 不信、疑惑

[l. 10] **substance use disorder:** 物質使用障害

[l. 34] **physiological:** 生理学上の

[l. 35] **withdrawal symptoms:** 禁断症状、離脱症状

[l. 44] **turn down:** 断る

☑Vocabulary Check

Match each word in the box with the most appropriate definition shown below.

Words	Definitions	Words	Definitions
problematic		divert	
evidence		nutrient	
craving		aversion	
drastically		impact	
overlap		partake	

Definitions:

a. a powerful desire for something

b. join in

c. cause to change course or turn from one direction to another

d. have an effect

e. radically, extremely

f. a substance that gives essential nutrition

g. presenting a problem

h. the available body of facts

i. cover shared parts of different subjects

j. a strong dislike

? Vocabulary Practice

Complete the following sentences with the words shown in the box. Change the grammatical form if necessary.

1. The economic growth of that country (   ) slowed.

2. The parents tried to (   ) their child's interest from TV games to study.

3. Students at the high school are to (   ) in some club activity.

4. My husband's work schedule (   ) with mine.

5. Some people have a strong (   ) to bull fighting.

6. Generally speaking, cabbage has lots of (   ).

7. This medicine is said to have caused (   ) behavior in some people who take it.

8. That terrible news had a big (   ) on people's minds.

9. There was sufficient (   ) that he was guilty.

10. After dinner, I tend to have a strong (   ) for chocolate.

✍ Comprehension

Read the following sentences on the content of the article and choose the best answer.

1. What do people with a substance use disorder continue doing?
>   **a.** They spend their money.
>   **b.** They get sick again and again.
>   **c.** They can't stop using a substance.
>   **d.** They take very good care of their health.

2. What sacrifice might people with substance dependence make?
>   **a.** They might stop some activities that previously brought them joy.
>   **b.** They might give a lot of money to charity.
>   **c.** They might change some bad habits to good ones.
>   **d.** They might not like to make their family happy.

3. What are two different symptoms of addiction?
>   **a.** Economic and occupational symptoms.
>   **b.** Social and psychological symptoms.
>   **c.** Personal and societal symptoms.
>   **d.** Physical and educational symptoms.

4. How can addiction affect a person's quality of living?
>   **a.** Quality of life can be partially improved.
>   **b.** Quality of life can be dramatically benefited.
>   **c.** Quality of life can be slightly denied.
>   **d.** Quality of life can be drastically reduced.

5. What is NOT listed as something affecting the signs and symptoms of substance use disorder?
>   **a.** Family history.
>   **b.** Personal circumstances.
>   **c.** Hobbies and interests.
>   **d.** Substance or behavior.

ⓘ Coffee Break

America's Deadly Sugar Addiction Has Reached Epidemic Levels

Americans are eating dessert three times a day—and they don't even know it. Sugar and other sweeteners are the main ingredients in some of America's favorite drinks and foods. And they've become ingrained in the American diet, considering the average American consumes about 20 teaspoons, or 80 grams, of sugar a day. The sweet stuff is a ubiquitous source of calories in the Western diet. However, now experts argue, sweeteners are contributors to major diseases.

Source: https://www.healthline.com/health/sugar/americas-deadly-sugar-addiction#1

🕮 Words & Phrases ─────────────────────────

ingrained: 深くしみ込んだ，変えがたい
ubiquitous: 遍在する、至る所にある

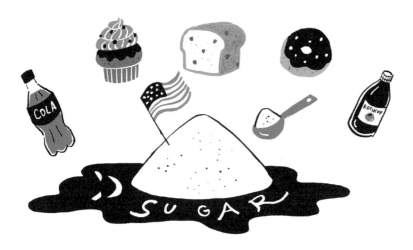

Unit 3

Virtual Reality Therapy

⌘Pre-reading⌘

　VR ゴーグルを装着すると、視界が 360 度覆われ、現在の居場所と全く異なる空間にいる感覚を得ることができ、現実に近い仮想の世界に身を置くことができます。今、ゲーム業界以外でも、スポーツトレーニング、デジタル広告や医療技術の開発など、様々な分野で VR 技術を応用する試みが広がっています。では、医療の分野で恐怖症治療における VR 技術の活用事例を見てみましょう。

⌘Reading⌘

12　Dick Tracey didn't have to visit a tall building to get over his fear of heights. He put on a virtual reality headset.

　Through VR, he rode an elevator to a high-rise atrium that looked so real he fell to his knees.

　"I needed to search with my hand for something solid around me," he 5 said.

　He told himself, "I must look stupid. Let's just stand up. Nothing's going to happen."

13　Virtual reality therapy can help people like Tracey by exposing them gradually to their greatest terrors. The technology is just now reaching the 10 mainstream after 20 years of research. Equipment is lighter and more affordable, with tech advances spilling over from the gaming industry to help people fight disabling fears of flying, heights, spiders or dogs.

　And the surge in products is bringing VR to more therapists' offices. Experts predict people with mild phobias will treat themselves successfully 15 at home.

　Research shows VR therapy can lead to real-world gains for people with phobias, and works as well as traditional exposure therapy, which slowly subjects patients to what causes anxiety for them.

14　For Denver librarian Nick Harrell, VR was a booster shot after tradi- 20 tional therapy for fear of flying. Panic drove him off a flight to Paris two years ago, forcing him to abandon a vacation with his girlfriend.

　"I don't like being locked in the metal tube," Harrell explained. "I couldn't breathe. My chest was pounding."

　With help from a therapist, Harrell first faced his fears through expo- 25 sure therapy. Elevators, buses and trains were good practice for airplanes.

"Within a matter of months, I was flying again," Harrell said.

With VR recently added to his therapy, Harrell keeps fears in check. His health insurance covers the cost with a small copay.

Mr. Tracey's VR therapy was part of a study. He was one of the first to 30 try a VR world with an animated virtual coach. University of Oxford psychology professor Daniel Freeman developed the program for an Oxford spin-off with support from the National Health Service.

Freeman's team is now at work on a VR world where people with schizophrenia can practice being in a cafe, elevator or store. 35

"Many of our patients are withdrawn from the world," Freeman said. The fear-of-heights VR program shows you can automate treatment.

What is VR? Put on a headset and look around. You'll see a simulation of an interactive, three-dimensional environment. Look up and you'll see the sky; look down and your own hands and feet may come into view. 40

With exposure therapy, a therapist can accompany a person who's afraid of heights to a tall building. With VR, a patient learns to feel safe on a virtual high-rise balcony, without leaving the therapist's office.

Exposure works by gradually taking the oomph out of panic. Sweaty palms and pounding hearts ease. Fears shrink to manageable levels. By rid- 45 ing it out, a person learns the feelings are survivable.

🗣 Words & Phrases

[l. 3] **a high-rise atrium:** 高層ビルのアトリウム（大規模な吹き抜け空間）

[l. 12] **spill over from A to B:** A から B に波及する

[l. 14] **surge in products:** 商品の急増

[l. 19] **subject somebody to〜:** 人を〜にさらす

[l. 20] **a booster shot:** 効果促進剤（比喩）

[l. 28] **keep fears in check:** 恐怖を抑えたままにする

[l. 29] **copay:** 医療費の支払いを患者が健康保険で一部まかなう事（= co-payment）

[l. 33] **spin-off:** スピンオフ。企業が事業部などの一部門を独立させて別の会社（例えば、子会社）を作ること

[l. 33] **National Health Service:** イギリスの国営医療サービス事業

[l. 34] **schizophrenia:** 統合失調症

[l. 44] **oomph:** 震え、活力、精力

[l. 45] **ride out:** 乗り切る

☑Vocabulary Check

Match each word in the box with the most appropriate definition shown below.

Words	Definitions	Words	Definitions
phobia		abandon	
affordable		withdraw	
spill		pound	
disable		shrink	
surge		manageable	

Definitions:

a. give up

b. strike or hit repeatedly

c. become smaller

d. a sudden large increase

e. easy to handle

f. remove or take away

g. prevent function or make unusable

h. an extreme fear

i. not expensive, or easy to purchase

j. fall out without plan

⚲ Vocabulary Practice

Complete the following sentences with the words shown in the box. Change the grammatical form if necessary.

1. The amount of work has been reduced so it is now (   ) for him.

2. Politicians in that country are trying to (   ) an unpopular leader.

3. She has a/an (   ) about being in a small, closed space.

4. "It is no use crying over (   ) milk."

5. The shirt (   ) after being machine-washed.

6. Unfortunately, he became (   ) in the car accident.

7. There was a/an (   ) in the population of Japan after World

War II.

8. Personal computers are now more (   ) than before.

9. During the festival in that village, people (   ) on a lot of different drums.

10. Fortunately, the troops from the neighboring countries have begun to
(   ).

✍ Comprehension

Choose the correct phrase to complete the sentence in line with the article.

1. The VR technology is just now (   ) after 20 years of research.
   a. beginning to work
   b. becoming widely known
   c. reaching completion
   d. showing good results

2. Experts predict people with mild phobias will treat themselves (   ).
   a. and damage their health
   b. in dental clinics
   c. better in the future
   d. on their own

3. With help from a therapist, Harrell (   ) through exposure therapy.
   a. dealt with what scared him
   b. learned to change his view
   c. became a better pilot
   d. wanted to take a vacation

4. Look up and you'll see the sky; look down and your own hands and feet
(   ).
   a. can grow to the size of trees
   b. might be visible
   c. might disappear from sight
   d. will look like wheels

5. Exposure (   ) taking the oomph out of panic.
   a. is famous for
   b. helps people enjoy
   c. looks fun while it is
   d. helps little by little by

ⓘ Coffee Break

Russian cows get VR headsets to reduce anxiety

A Russian farm has given its dairy cows virtual reality headsets in a bid to reduce their anxiety. Moscow's Ministry of Agriculture and Food cited research which they say has shown a link between a cow's emotional experience and its milk production. Initial tests reportedly boosted the overall emotional mood of the herd. According to a statement from the ministry, examples of dairy farms from different countries show that in a calm atmosphere, the quantity, and sometimes the quality, of milk increases markedly. Researchers will examine the effects of the program in a long-term study. The developers hope to expand the project if positive results continue.

Source: https://www.bbc.com/news/world-europe-50571010

☰ Words & Phrases ────────────────────

dairy cow: 乳牛
in a bid to: ～しょうとして
cite: （例証の為に）～に言及する
reportedly: 報道によると
herd: 群れ
markedly: 著しく
Moscows Ministry of Agriculture and Food: モスクワ農業食糧省

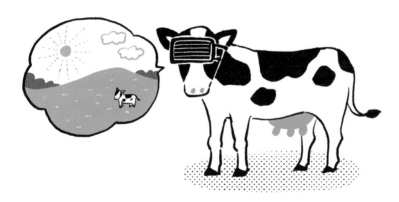

☺ Useful Expressions 1

At the Drug Store

Store Staff: Hello. How can I help you?

Customer: Hi. I'm looking for
headache medicine.
indigestion medicine.
sea-sick medicine.
pain relievers.
dietary supplements.
vitamin supplements.

Store Staff: Okay, they are
over here.
on aisle three.

Customer: What are the active ingredients in this one?

Store Staff: This one contains diphenhydramine.

Customer: Does it cause drowsiness?

Store Staff: Yes, it does. So, you shouldn't drive if you use it.

Customer: Do you have any
herbal medicines?
alternative medications?

Store Staff: We have some Chinese medicines, called KAMPO.

Customer: What are they made of?

Store Staff: Most of them are plant-based remedies.

Customer: Do they have any side-effects?

Store Staff: No, the ones that we sell have no side-effects.

Customer: Thank you. I'll try this one.

🐚 Words & Phrases

indigestion medicine: 消化不良治療薬
pain relievers: 痛み止め
dietary supplements: 栄養補助食品
aisle: 商店などの通路
active ingredient: 活性要素、有効成分
diphenhydramine: ジフェンヒドラミン（抗ヒスタミン薬）
drowsiness: 眠気
herbal medicines: 漢方薬
alternative medications:（テキストの会話の場合）他の薬、代替薬品
remedies: 医療品・治療（法）
side-effects: 副作用

🖧 Let's check !

Common Medication Forms（よく見る薬の形状）

pill
hard capsule
soft capsule
enteric coated tablet
syrup
drop
powder
ointment
vial
troche
spray
inhalant

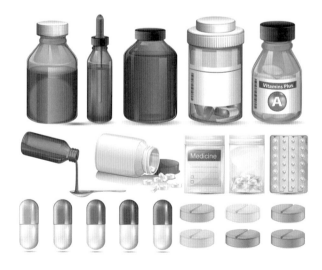

Unit 4

Back Pain

⌘Pre-reading⌘

　腰痛の原因がいくつかあります。それらを探り、いつ医者にかかればいいのか、またその予防法などを読みます。長時間立っている場合や、歩き続けた後の痛みはしばらく座れば楽になる場合もあります。様々な鎮痛剤や軽い運動で痛みが緩和されることもありますが、手術という選択肢もあります。

⌘Reading⌘

Causes of lower back pain when standing or walking

Lower back pain is very common, so determining an underlying cause may often come down to looking at other symptoms and details. If lower back pain occurs when standing or walking, the pain may be due to muscle fatigue. 5

In this article, we look at some potential causes of lower back pain that occur when standing or walking. We also cover when to see a doctor and some prevention tips.

Muscle fatigue

Rest may help relieve lower back pain. Prolonged walking or standing 10 can tire or strain the muscles in the lower back and legs, which can lead to aches and pains. This pain or discomfort usually gets better with sitting or lying down to rest the back. People who are overweight may be more at risk for muscle fatigue that occurs when standing or walking.

Treatment 15

A person can treat muscle fatigue and reduce discomfort in the lower back with:

- rest
- hot or cold therapy
- over-the-counter (OTC) pain relievers, such as ibuprofen and naproxen 20
- gentle exercises to stretch and loosen tight muscles

Maintaining a healthy weight can also help reduce stress on the back and legs.

Lumbar spinal stenosis

Spinal stenosis is a narrowing of the spine that can place extra pressure 25 on the spinal cord and nerves. Spinal stenosis often occurs in the lower part of the back, or lumbar spine, where it can lead to lower back pain when walking or standing. People often find that this pain improves with sitting down or leaning forward.

Other symptoms of lumbar spinal stenosis can include: 30

- weakness in the legs
- numbness or tingling in the lower back, buttocks, or legs
- sciatica, or sharp pain that radiates down the leg

Severe spinal stenosis may lead to bowel and bladder problems and sexual dysfunction. Spinal stenosis usually occurs as a result of aging and is 35 most common in people over the age of 50 years. However, some people are born with a narrow spinal canal, and spinal stenosis can also develop following a spinal injury.

Treatment

A doctor may first recommend nonsurgical treatments for people with 40 spinal stenosis. The options may include:

- physical therapy
- nonsteroidal anti-inflammatory drugs (NSAIDs), such as ibuprofen or naproxen
- steroid injections 45
- alternative therapies, such as chiropractic treatment or acupuncture

If a person's pain worsens or does not improve, a doctor may recommend a surgical procedure to stabilize the spine or relieve pressure on the spinal nerves.

🦪 Words & Phrases

[l. 20] **over-the-counter (OTC):** 市販の
[l. 20] **ibuprofen:** イブプロフェン。プロピオン酸系に分類されるステロイド系消炎鎮痛剤の一種
[l. 20] **naproxen:** ナプロキセン。芳香族カルボン酸に分類される有機化合物で鎮痛、解熱、抗炎症薬として用いられる非ステロイド性抗炎症薬の一種
[l. 24] **lumbar spinal stenosis:** 腰部脊柱管狭窄症
[l. 26] **spinal cord:** 脊髄
[l. 27] **lumbar spine:** 腰椎
[l. 32] **numbness:** 無感覚
[l. 32] **tingle:** ひりひり，うずうず，きりきり痛む
[l. 33] **sciatica:** 座骨神経痛

[l. 37]　**spinal canal:** 脊椎菅
[l. 43]　**nonsteroidal anti-inflammatory drugs:** 非ステロイド系抗炎症薬
[l. 46]　**chiropractic treatment:** カイロプラクティック、脊柱指圧療法
[l. 46]　**acupuncture:** 鍼（はり）療法

☑Vocabulary Check

Match each word in the box with the most appropriate definition shown below.

Words	Definitions	Words	Definitions
underlying		discomfort	
fatigue		radiate	
numb		alternative	
prolong		worsen	
strain		relieve	

Definitions:

a. make it last longer
b. make something do more than it is able to do
c. spread from a central point
d. extreme tiredness
e. unable to feel anything in a particular part of your body
f. hidden or not clear
g. painful feeling in part of your body
h. to take away or lessen
i. becomes more difficult or unpleasant
j. something that is different from the usual things of its kind

♀ Vocabulary Practice

Complete the following sentences with the words shown in the box. Change the grammatical form if necessary.

　1. One of the symptoms of this illness is extreme (　　　　　　　　).

　2. The bad relationship between country A and country B has been
　　 (　　　　　　　) because of corruption.

3. I was (   ) when I finally saw my son's face at the front door.

4. His back pain (   ), lasting for a much longer period than he imagined.

5. Her face (   ) with joy, when she heard the news.

6. What principle was (   ) his hostile action against the government?

7. She (   ) her leg muscle when climbing the stairs..

8. I was lying in a weird position and my leg went (   ).

9. When the train is delayed, you have to find a/an (   ) form of transportation.

10. "Do you feel any (   ) somewhere in your body?" "No, not really."

✍ Comprehension

Underline the words in each sentence that don't match the content of the article and correct them.

1. Determining a necessary response may often come down to looking at other symptoms and details.

   ⇒ (   )

2. The artide also covers when to see a doctor and some helpful cures.

   ⇒ (   )

3. People who are overweight may like to enjoy exercising for muscle fatigue that occurs when standing or walking.

   ⇒ (   )

4. Spinal stenosis never affects areas below the lower part of the back, or lumbar spine.

   ⇒ (   )

5. If a person's pain worsens or does not improve, a patient can easily request a surgical procedure.

   ⇒ (   )

ⓘ Coffee Break

Back Pain Risk Factors

Anyone can develop back pain, even children and teens. These factors might put you at greater risk of developing back pain.

- ☐ **Age:** Back pain is more common as you get older, starting around age 30 or 40.

- ☐ **Lack of exercise:** Weak, unused muscles in your back and abdomen might lead to back pain.

- ☐ **Excess weight:** Excess body weight puts extra stress on your back.

- ☐ **Diseases:** Some types of arthritis and cancer can contribute to back pain.

- ☐ **Improper lifting:** Using your back instead of your legs can lead to back pain.

- ☐ **Psychological conditions:** People prone to depression and anxiety appear to have a greater risk of back pain.

- ☐ **Smoking:** This reduces blood flow to the lower spine, which can keep your body from delivering enough nutrients to the disks in your back. Smoking also slows healing.

Source: https://www.mayoclinic.org/diseases-conditions/back-pain/symptoms-causes/syc

🕮 Words & Phrases

arthritis: 関節炎
be prone to〜: 〜の傾向がある
disk: 椎間板

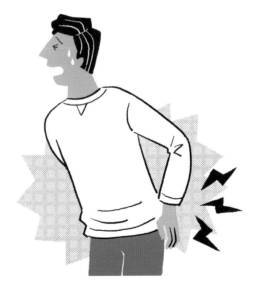

Unit 5

Risky Aspirin?

⌘Pre-reading⌘

　アスピリンは、アセチルサリチル酸でドイツの製薬会社バイエルが名付けた商標名なのです。熱や痛みなどの症状を抑えます。アメリカでは人々は簡単にこの薬品を手に入れ、常備薬としてよく使います。解熱や頭痛の改善などの目的以外に、心臓発作や脳卒中を防ぐ効果があると信じて、毎日アスピリンを服用するアメリカ人もいます。しかし、最近の研究によると、もともと健康な人が服用すると、利点よりも健康被害を受ける可能性があることがわかりました。

⌘Reading⌘

For people without heart disease, taking a daily aspirin to prevent heart attacks and strokes may increase the risk of severe brain bleeding to the point where it outweighs any potential benefit, a research review suggests.

U.S. doctors have long advised adults who haven't had a heart attack or stroke but are at high risk for these events to take a daily aspirin pill, an 5 approach known as primary prevention. Even though there's clear evidence aspirin works for this purpose, many physicians and patients have been reluctant to follow the recommendations because of the risk of rare but potentially lethal internal bleeding.

For the current study, researchers examined data from 13 clinical trials 10 testing the effects of aspirin against a placebo or no treatment in more than 134,000 adults.

The risk of intracranial hemorrhage, or brain bleeds, was rare: taking aspirin was associated with two additional cases of this type of internal bleeding for every 1,000 people, the study found.　　　　　　　　　　　15

But the bleeding risk was still 37 percent higher for people taking aspirin than for people who didn't take this drug.

"Intracranial hemorrhage is a special concern because it is strongly associated with a high risk of death and poorer health over a lifetime," said study co-author Dr. Meng Lee of Chang Gung University College of Med- 20 icine in Taiwan.

"These findings suggest caution regarding using low-dose aspirin in individuals without symptomatic cardiovascular disease," Lee said by email.

For people who have already had a heart attack or stroke, the benefit of low-dose aspirin to prevent another major cardiac event is well estab- 25 lished, researchers note in JAMA Neurology. But the value of aspirin is less clear for healthier people, for whom bleeding risks may outweigh any benefit.

For adults ages 50 to 59 considering aspirin to prevent heart attacks and strokes, for example, the U.S Preventive Services Task Force (USPSTF) 30 recommends the pill only for people who have at least a 10 percent risk of having a heart attack or stroke over the next decade and who don't have a higher-than-average risk of bleeding.

One limitation of the analysis is that the smaller clinical trials examined a variety of aspirin doses up to 100 milligrams daily. The analysis also only 35 focused on brain bleeds, and not on other types of internal bleeding associated with aspirin.

"We have long known that aspirin can precipitate bleeding, most commonly in the gastrointestinal tract, but most devastatingly in the brain," said Dr. Samuel Wann, a cardiologist at Ascension Healthcare in Milwau- 40 kee, Wisconsin, who wasn't involved in the study.

Despite the benefits for preventing heart attacks, the consensus on aspirin has changed over time, particularly for people without heart disease or hardening and narrowing of the arteries (atherosclerosis).

🐾 Words & Phrases

[l. 2]   **stroke:** 脳卒中
[l. 11]   **placebo:** 気休めの薬。薬効はないが、実験的・臨床的に試験する時の対照薬
[l. 13]   **intracranial hemorrhage:** 頭蓋内出血、脳出血
[l. 20]   **Chang Gung University College of Medicine in Taiwan:** 長庚大学(台湾の私立大学) 医学部
[l. 23]   **symptomatic cardiovascular disease:** 症候性心血管疾患
[l. 26]   **JAMA Neurology:** アメリカ医学会により出版されている神経学系月刊誌
[l. 30]   **U.S Preventive Services Task Force (USPSTF):** アメリカ合衆国予防医療専門委員会
[l. 39]   **gastrointestinal tract:** 消化器官
[l. 40]   **Ascension Healthcare in Milwaukee:** ミルウォーキー市アセンションヘルスケアセンター
[l. 44]   **atherosclerosis:** アテローム性動脈硬化

☑Vocabulary Check

Match each word in the box with the most appropriate definition shown below.

Words	Definitions	Words	Definitions
outweigh		cardiac	
benefit		dose	
reluctant		precipitate	
lethal		devastatingly	
concern		consensus	

Definitions:

a. very destructive or damaging

b. likely to cause death

c. unwilling and hesitant

d. a general agreement

e. cause to happen suddenly

f. an advantage or profit

g. a quantity of a medicine taken at one time

h. anxiety, worry

i. relating to the heart

j. be greater or heavier

♀ Vocabulary Practice

Complete the following sentences with the words shown in the box. Change the grammatical form if necessary.

1. The Congress finally reached a/an (   ).

2. The powerful typhoon hit the area with (   ) force.

3. He grabbed his chest when he suffered from a/an (   ) arrest.

4. Both sides get (   ) from this business deal.

5. Some people die after taking a/an (   ) amount of sleeping pills.

6. He (   ) agreed to the plan.

7. You have to always keep in mind the (   ) of the medicine when taking it.

8. Global warming is a/an (   ) for the leaders of every country in the world.

9. The advantages of this method far (   ) the others.

10. The outbreak of the terrible epidemic (   ) the country's economic decline.

✍ Comprehension

Read the following sentences on the content of the article and choose the best answer.

1. What is a danger of taking an aspirin pill every day.
    a. It can prevent regular headaches.
    b. It can cause a stroke or heart attack.
    c. It can increase the risk of severe brain bleeding.
    d. It can accelerate the speed of primary prevention.

2. How much higher is the risk for people who take aspirin than for people who didn't?
    a. The risk was not much higher.
    b. The risk was 37% higher.
    c. The risk was worth the danger.
    d. The risk was unknown but slightly higher.

3. Who can most clearly benefit from taking a daily dose of aspirin?
    a. People who have already had a heart attack or stroke most benefit.
    b. Researchers find that everyone can benefit equally.
    c. People who want to have a brain bleed are the only ones who benefit.
    d. No one benefits because researchers have said that aspirin is so dangerous.

4. What is a limitation about the research study explained in the article? It didn't...
    a. give people enough aspirin to understand how much is dangerous.
    b. check if other areas of the body are damaged by heart attacks.
    c. ask enough researchers to join the study and help.
    d. examine other types of internal bleeding associated with aspirin.

5. What does "the consensus on aspirin has changed over time" mean?

    a. All medical experts agree that aspirin is only useful for headaches.

    b. How most doctors think about aspirin is different now than in the past.

    c. People don't agree with what medical experts say about aspirin.

    d. Aspirin is a safe drug that everyone agrees needs to be used carefully.

ⓘ Coffee Break

What is aspirin?

Aspirin is one of the most widely used medications in the world. It comes from salicylate, which can be found in plants such as willow trees and myrtle. It is a non-steroidal anti-inflammatory drug.

Non-steroidal means they are not steroids. Steroids often have similar benefits, but they can have unwanted side effects.

Aspirin in its present form has been around for over 100 years. It is still one of the most widely used medications in the world. It is estimated that around 35,000 metric tons of aspirin are consumed annually.

Aspirin is a trademark owned by the German pharmaceutical company, Bayer. The generic term for aspirin is acetylsalicylic acid (ASA).

Source: https://www.medicalnewstoday.com/articles/161255.php

🕮 Words & Phrases

salicylate: サリチル酸塩
willow: 柳
myrtle: ギンバイカ（銀梅花）
non-steroidal: 非ステロイド性の
anti-inflammatory: 抗炎症の
metric ton: メートル法のトン
generic term: 一般名称
acetylsalicylic acid:
アセチルサリチル酸（ASA）

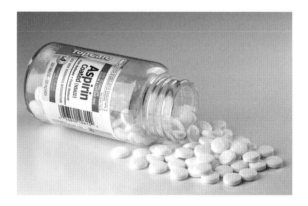

Unit 6

New Trends in Controlling Cancer

⌘Pre-reading⌘

現在日本は、ほぼ3人に1人はがんで亡くなる時代だと言われています。早期発見、早期治療によって、がんの進行を抑えることは可能ですが、がんは非常に治りにくい病気です。外科療法、放射線療法及び抗がん剤などによる化学療法は、標準的な治療法として実践されていますが、それぞれに一長一短があって決定的なものはまだ見つかっていません。がん治療の現場で、日々新たな研究と開発が行われています。将来への期待として確立されつつある治療法について読んでいきましょう。

⌘Reading⌘

 There's good news for cancer patients: Treatments are becoming less invasive and taking less time.

Traditional treatments often include chemotherapy or radiation to kill cancer cells and shrink tumors. The treatments kill healthy cells as well as cancerous ones, and the side effects are legendary. 5

Surgery can be an option, too. Sometimes it's all that's needed, but many people have some combination of chemo, radiation and surgery. These treatments can span months, and patients have months more of recovery time.

 Cancer treatment is now moving toward precision medicine that targets 10 just the cancer.

For example, doctors are using focused radiation, after a lumpectomy, for women who have early stage breast cancer. With this procedure, radiation beams pinpoint the tumor from hundreds of different angles for a short period of time. Each beam itself is weak, but together, when they hit 15 the tumor, the result is a higher dose of radiation.

Dr. Julia White at the Ohio State University Comprehensive Cancer Center found focused radiation has the same positive results as full breast radiation. Plus, the partial radiation takes only five days.

White said, "The short five-day treatment is just as good as the whole 20 breast irradiation that lasts for four to six weeks."

 Other treatments use the body's own immune system. Dr. William Nelson at Johns Hopkins Medicine told VOA it's clear that the immune system sees cancer cells as abnormal, "and if we unleash the immune system, it can attack and destroy the cancer cells." 25

The American Cancer Society says immunotherapy has become an important part of treating some cancers, and that newer types of immune treatments, currently being studied, will affect how we treat cancer in the future.

Still another new treatment, genomic testing, involves testing the cancer 30 cells to determine their genetic makeup.

Most cancers start because of genetic mutations, and each patient's cancer is unique, just like his or her DNA. If doctors know the particular DNA, they can prescribe medicine that targets the mutated cells. Healthy cells are left alone. And few patients have any side effects. If they do, the 35 doctor lowers the dose of the medication. It eliminates the side effect, and the treatment is still effective.

Because genomic testing is so costly, the biggest impact right now is for patients whose cancer keeps returning or spreads to other parts of the body. That's why it isn't seen as a first-line treatment yet. But the results 40 are outstanding.

Cancer specialists think targeted therapy, immunotherapy or genomic testing and precision medicine are the future of cancer treatment. And one day, it will be the standard treatment worldwide.

📖 Words & Phrases ━━━━━━━━━━━━━━━━━━━━━━━━━━━━

[l. 5] **cancerous:** がんにかかった

[l. 10] **precision medicine:** 精密医療

[l. 12] **lumpectomy:** 腫瘍摘出手術

[l. 17] **Ohio State University Comprehensive Cancer Center:** オハイオ州立大学付属総合がんセンター

[l. 23] **Johns Hopkins Medicine:** ジョンズ・ホプキンズ病院。アメリカ合衆国メリーランド州ボルチモアに位置する、ジョンズ・ホプキンズ大学医学部附属の教育病院・生物医学研究施設。1889 年設立

[l. 26] **American Cancer Society:** アメリカがん協会　https://www.vancer.org/

[l. 26] **immunotherapy:** 免疫療法

[l. 30] **genomic test:** ゲノム検査

[l. 31] **genetic makeup:** 遺伝子構造

[l. 40] **first-line treatment**: 第一線（第一選択）治療

☑Vocabulary Check

Match each word in the box with the most appropriate definition shown below.

Words	Definitions	Words	Definitions
invasive		unleash	
tumor		genetic	
legendary		mutate	
chemotherapy		prescribe	
abnormal		eliminate	

Definitions:

a. to develop new physical characteristics because of a permanent change in the genes

b. different from what is usual or average, especially in a bad way

c. extensive, aggressive or causing great effect

d. a type of treatment that uses chemicals to kill harmful, cancerous cells and prevent them from reproducing

e. relating to parts of the DNA in cells received by each animal or plant from its parents

f. a mass of harmful cells in the body that grow faster than usual and can cause illness

g. extremely well-known, greater in degree than the usual

h. to release a powerful force that cannot be controlled

i. to remove or take away someone or something

j. to say what medical treatment a patient should have

⚲ Vocabulary Practice

Complete the following sentences with the words shown in the box. Change the grammatical form if necessary.

1. The doctor (   ) some strong pain killers and told her to drink more water.

2. The atmosphere in the classroom was casual and friendly, which helped students (   ) their ideas and imagination.

3. She made a full recovery after she had a/an (   ) removed from her stomach.

4. Everyone knew that he smoked like a chimney and his drinking was even more ( ).

5. ( ) testing uses laboratory methods to look at your DNA information to identify increased risks of health problems.

6. The TV news announced that a/an ( ) level of radiation had been recorded in this area.

7. ( ) acts on the whole body, and it's particularly effective for treating rapidly spreading cancers.

8. Although it is possible to keep this virus from being active, it is very difficult to ( ) it entirely from the body.

9. Cancer is considered a/an ( ) disease because it can get out of control and spread from one organ to another.

10. Because more people are getting infected and showing more severe symptoms, the virus may have ( ) into a more powerful form.

✍ Comprehension

Choose the correct phrase to complete the sentence in line with the article.

1. The traditional treatments kill healthy cells ( ), and the side effects are legendary.

    a. in addition to malignant cells
    b. instead of healing the body
    c. in order to destroy the illness
    d. because they are dangerous

2. Cancer treatment is ( ) precision medicine that targets just the cancer.

    a. famous for being a
    b. useful when it is
    c. currently developing
    d. trying to find a new

3. Each radiation beam itself is weak, but together, when they hit the tumor, the ( ) dose of radiation.

    a. energy reduces the
    b. outcome is a larger
    c. cancer is destroyed by the low
    d. patient can strongly feel a

4. Immunotherapy has become (   ) treating some cancers.
    a. a valued element in
    b. a profitable way for
    c. fun for people who are
    d. the best method for

5. Genomic testing (   ) cells to determine their genetic makeup.
    a. is a way to measure
    b. gives a complex medication to
    c. is done by examining cancer
    d. releases chemicals into

ⓘ Coffee Break

Eat Healthy and Get Active

Although our genes influence our risk of cancer, most of the difference in cancer risk between people is due to factors that are not inherited. Avoiding tobacco products, staying at a healthy weight, staying active throughout life, and eating a healthy diet may greatly reduce a person's lifetime risk of developing or dying from cancer. These same behaviors are also linked with a lower risk of developing heart disease and diabetes.

Source: https://www.cancer.org/

☲ Words & Phrases ────────────────────────────────

inherit: ～を遺伝で受け継ぐ

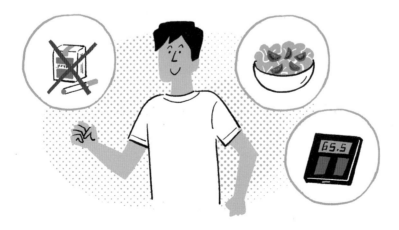

☺ Useful Expressions 2

At the Pharmacy

Pharmacist: Hello, Mr. Williams.
These are the medications your doctor has prescribed for

your	headache.
	dizziness.
	upset stomach.
	infection.
	high blood pressure.

You should take	one tablet,	two times per day.
		on a full stomach.
	two capsules,	mornings and evenings.
		for seven days.
	200 milligrams	after meals.

Customer: Thank you. Does this medicine have any side-effects?

Pharmacist: Yes, sometimes. You might feel

some	nausea.
mild	bloating.
occasional	drowsiness.
	gas.
	burping.
	heart burn.
	diarrhea.
	trouble sleeping.
	blurred vision.
	headaches.
	nose bleeds.

If you have any strong reactions, please contact	us.
	your doctor.

Customer: Okay. What is the dosage of this drug?

Pharmacist: It's 125 milligrams per tablet. (125mg / tab).

Customer: While taking this, is it okay to | drink alcohol?
drive?
take my heart medicine?
take vitamins?

Pharmacist: Yes, It's okay.
No, you shouldn't
I'm not sure. Please ask your doctor.

Customer: Do I need to see my doctor to refill this prescription?

Pharmacist: No, you can just come back here.
Yes, you need a new prescription from a doctor.

🕮 Words & Phrases

dizziness:（フラフラする）目まい
upset stomach: 胃のむかつき
infection: 感染
high blood pressure: 高血圧
on a full stomach: 食後
nausea: 吐き気
bloating: 膨満感
burping: げっぷ
ringing in one's ears:（両耳で起きる）耳鳴り
heart burn: 胸やけ
diarrhea: 下痢
trouble sleeping: 不眠
blurred vision: かすみ目
nose bleeds: 鼻血
dosage: 投薬量、服用量
refill: 補充する
prescription: 処方箋　☞ to refill a prescription: 再調剤する

Unit 7

Hyaluronic Acid

⌘Pre-reading⌘

　ヒアルロン酸は、私たちの眼や関節部分に多く存在しています。保湿作用があるので化粧品によく使われていることはご存じでしょう。現在では膝の障害の治療、眼の病気の手術だけでなく、美容整形にも使われます。このように広く使用されていると、その安全性を見落としがちになりますが、安全であると実証されていないケースも存在するので注意が必要です。

⌘Reading⌘

Hyaluronic acid is a substance that is naturally present in the human body. It is found in the highest concentrations in fluids in the eyes and joints. The hyaluronic that is used as medicine is extracted from rooster combs or made by bacteria in the laboratory.

People take hyaluronic acid for various joint disorders, including osteoarthritis. It can be taken by mouth or injected into the affected joint by a healthcare professional. 5

The FDA has approved the use of hyaluronic acid during certain eye surgeries including cataract removal, corneal transplantation, and repair of a detached retina and other eye injuries. It is injected into the eye during the procedure to help replace natural fluids. 10

Hyaluronic acid is also used as a lip filler in plastic surgery.

Some people apply hyaluronic acid to the skin for healing wounds, burns, skin ulcers, and as a moisturizer.

There is also a lot of interest in using hyaluronic acid to prevent the effects of aging. In fact, hyaluronic acid has been promoted as a "fountain of youth." However, there is no evidence to support the claim that taking it by mouth or applying it to the skin can prevent changes associated with aging. 15

How does it work? 20

Hyaluronic acid works by acting as a cushion and lubricant in the joints and other tissues. In addition, it might affect the way the body responds to injury.

Uses & effectiveness

Likely Effective for: 25

Cataracts. Injecting hyaluronic acid into the eye is effective when used during cataract surgery by an eye surgeon.

Sores in the mouth. Hyaluronic acid is effective for treating mouth sores when applied to the skin as a gel.

🎧35 Insufficient evidence for:

₃₀

Dry eye. Early research shows that applying a specific hyaluronic acid eye drop (Hyalistil) might relieve dry eye.

Eye trauma. Some research suggests that hyaluronic acid might be injected into the eye to treat detached retina or other eye injuries.

Healing skin wounds and burns. Early research suggests that applying ₃₅ hyaluronic acid to the skin might be helpful for treating burns and skin wounds.

More evidence is needed to rate the effectiveness of hyaluronic acid for these uses.

🎧36 Side Effects & Safety

₄₀

Hyaluronic acid is LIKELY SAFE when taken by mouth, applied to the skin, or given by injection. Rarely, hyaluronic acid may cause allergic reactions.

Special Precautions & Warnings

Pregnancy and breast-feeding: Hyaluronic acid is POSSIBLY SAFE when ₄₅ given by injection during pregnancy. However, not enough is known about the safety of hyaluronic acid when taken by mouth or applied to the skin during pregnancy. Stay on the safe side and avoid use.

Hyaluronic acid is POSSIBLY UNSAFE when given by injection during breast feeding.

₅₀

🗣 Words & Phrases ━━━━━━━━━━━━━━━━━━━━━━━━━━━━━━━━━━━━━

[l. 1] **hyaluronic acid:** ヒアルロン酸
[l. 3] **rooster comb**: 鶏のとさか
[l. 5] **osteoarthritis:** 変形性関節症
[l. 8] **FDA =Food and Drug Administration:** アメリカ食品医薬品局
[l. 9] **cataract:** 白内障、水晶体白濁の部位
[l. 9] **corneal:** 角膜
[l. 10] **detached retina:** 網膜剥離
[l. 12] **plastic surgery:** 美容外科
[l. 14] **skin ulcer:** 皮膚潰瘍
[l. 32] **Hyalistil:** ヒアルロン酸点眼薬
[l. 33] **eye trauma:** 眼の外傷

☑Vocabulary Check

Match each word in the box with the most appropriate definition shown below.

Words	Definitions	Words	Definitions
approve		lubricant	
detach		sore	
apply		rate	
promote		side effect	
associate		precaution	

Definitions:

a. an action taken in advance to prevent something dangerous

b. evaluate and rank the value of something

c. a secondary effect of a drug or medical treatment

d. a painful place on the body

e. put or spread on a surface

f. agree or accept

g. leave or separate from

h. a substance used to make parts move smoothly

i. try to increase the popularity of

j. connect, relate

♀ Vocabulary Practice

Complete the following sentences with the words shown in the box. Change the grammatical form if necessary.

1. Small talk could be a/an (   ) for making good relations among people.

2. My friend's speech was (   ) the highest in our English class.

3. This cold medicine is (   ) on TV as effective.

4. Because of the terrible (   ) in my mouth, I can hardly eat anything.

5. The marathon runner (   ) himself from the main group on the last lap.

6. This Japanese automobile company is (　　　　　　　) with that German company.

7. Is there any (　　　　　　　) caused by this injection against influenza?

8. The new medicine was recently (　　　　　　　) by the Ministry of Health and Welfare.

9. What kind of (　　　　　　　) is necessary when climbing Mt. Fuji?

10. (　　　　　　　) this moisturizing cream to you skin after bathing or showering.

✍ Comprehension

Underline the words in each sentence that don't match the content of the article and correct them.

1. Hyaluronic acid can be inhaled as a steam or injected into the affected joint by a healthcare professional.

⇒ (　　　　　　　　　　　　　　　　　　　　　　　　　　　)

2. Some people apply hyaluronic acid to the skin for healing wounds, burns, skin ulcers, and to improve health.

⇒ (　　　　　　　　　　　　　　　　　　　　　　　　　　　)

3. There is no evidence to explain the fact that taking it by mouth or applying it to the skin can prevent changes associated with aging.

⇒ (　　　　　　　　　　　　　　　　　　　　　　　　　　　)

4. Some research suggests that hyaluronic acid might be injected into the eye to treat detached retina or change your eye color.

⇒ (　　　　　　　　　　　　　　　　　　　　　　　　　　　)

5. Not enough is known about the safety of hyaluronic acid when taken by mouth or applied after being in the sun.

⇒ (　　　　　　　　　　　　　　　　　　　　　　　　　　　)

ⓘ Coffee Break

Is Hyaluronic Acid Bad for Your Skin?

Hyaluronic acid (HA) is a type of molecule naturally found in your skin that pulls water from the air and sucks it into your face like a sponge, helping your skin stay moist throughout the day. Because of its ability to retain water, you'll also find it in a lot of makeup and hydrating skincare products.

Hyaluronic acid is great for your skin—when used and applied correctly and in the right order. Here's the deal: If your dry skin is sitting in a humid room and you slather on hyaluronic acid, it'll pull moisture from the air and into your dry face. But—but! —if your moisturized skin is sitting in a *dry* room during winter or in a dry climate, the hyaluronic acid sitting on top of your face will pull water *out* of your skin and evaporate it into the air, leaving your face drier than before. So ideally, after applying hyaluronic acid to your slightly damp skin, remember to top it off with a layer of face oil before bed to maximize the hydration.

Source: https://www.cosmopolitan.com/style-beauty/beauty/a32080573/
what-is-hyaluronic-acid-benefits-for-skin/

📖 Words & Phrases

molecule: 微粒子
moist: 湿った、しっとりとした
hydrating skincare products: 保湿用のスキンケア商品
moisture: （大気中に拡散した）水分
moisturized: 保湿された
slather on: 〜をたっぷりと塗る
evaporate: 〜を蒸発させる
damp: 湿気のある
top off with: 〜で終える、
〜で締めくくる
hydration: 水分補給

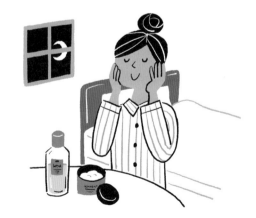

Unit 8

A Promising Treatment for Alzheimer's

⌘Pre-reading⌘

アルツハイマー型認知症は、脳が委縮していく病気で、病気が進行していくにつれて徐々に記憶力や判断力を失います。この認知能力の低下とともに意思の疎通ができなくなり、日常生活に様々な障害が生じて最終的には寝たきりになります。高齢化社会の日本では、アルツハイマー型認知症の患者数は年々増加する傾向にあります。しかしながら、病気の進行を遅らせたり、症状を緩和させたりする治療が中心で、病気を完全に治す治療法はまだ確立していません。

⌘Reading⌘

Dementia is a rapidly growing public health problem around the world. Fifty million people suffer from dementia, and in the next 30 years that number is expected to triple.

Researchers are looking for ways to treat or prevent dementia, and a promising clinical trial is underway in the U.S. 5

Dementia is not a normal part of aging, but age is a huge risk factor. Regular exercise, a healthy diet, maintaining healthy blood pressure, cholesterol, and blood sugar levels help stave off dementia as we grow older.

As people around the world live longer, health agencies and researchers are looking for ways to prevent, stop or treat dementia, including 10 Alzheimer's disease, one of the most common types of dementia.

Promising clinical trial

David Shorr was diagnosed with Alzheimer's at 56. He is about to undergo a new procedure that could treat early stage Alzheimer's. He is with his doctor, Vibhor Krishna, a neurosurgeon at Ohio State Wexner Medical 15 Center.

The procedure Shorr is about to have involves sound waves. Ultrasound waves target and open the blood-brain barrier — a protective layer that shields the brain from infections. But Krishna says the barrier also makes it hard to treat neurodegenerative diseases like Alzheimer's. 20

"Opening the blood-brain barrier allows us to access more of the brain tissue and be able to increase the effectiveness or bioavailability of the therapeutics," Krishna said.

Shorr and his wife, Kim, were willing to try any new treatment that might help with his dementia. Kim describes the couple's reaction when they received a phone call inviting Shorr to participate in a clinical trial.

"There's this trial. Would you be interested?" she said, describing the call. "And without really knowing what it was, we said, 'Sure'."

Ultrasound targets protein buildup

Shorr became one of 10 patients enrolled in the study. The trial tests MRI-guided imaging to target the part of the brain responsible for memory and cognition. Krishna explains that area is where Alzheimer's patients have a buildup of toxic proteins called amyloid.

"Higher deposition of amyloid goes hand in hand with loss of function in Alzheimer's disease," he said.

Krishna says this procedure might allow a patient's own immune system to clear some of the amyloid.

In this procedure, ultrasound wave pulses cause microscopic bubbles to expand and contract in the brain.

"The increase and decrease in size of these microbubbles mechanically opens the blood-brain barrier," Krishna said.

Opening the barrier may one day allow doctors to deliver medication straight to the site of the disease.

🎧 Words & Phrases

[l. 5] **clinical trial:** 臨床試験
[l. 9] **health agency:** 健康機関
[l. 15] **neurosurgeon:** 神経外科医
[l. 15] **Ohio State Wexner Medical Center:** オハイオ州立大学の付属病院（U.S. News & World Report の全米ベスト病院ランキング 2019-2020 年では耳鼻科、腫瘍内科、糖尿内分泌内科及び腎臓内科の四つの部門でランクインしている）
[l. 17] **ultrasound wave:** 超音波
[l. 18] **blood-brain barrier:** 血液脳関門
[l. 20] **neurodegenerative:** 神経変性の
[l. 22] **bioavailability of the therapeutics:** 治療法の生体利用効率
[l. 31] **MRI:** 磁気共鳴映像法（Magnetic Resonance Imaging）
[l. 33] **amyloid:** アミロイド（脳内で作られるたんぱく質の一種、アミロイドの異常な蓄積が認知症の原因とされている）

☑Vocabulary Check

Match each word in the box with the most appropriate definition shown below.

Words	Definitions	Words	Definitions
dementia		procedure	
underway		shield	
stave off		toxic	
diagnose		go hand in hand	
undergo		medication	

Definitions:

a. poisonous, or causing you a lot of harm over a long period of time

b. to experience something that is unpleasant but necessary

c. a medical condition causing memory and other mental abilities to become worse

d. to protect someone or something from harmful events or bad experiences

e. to recognize the exact character of a disease or a problem by making an examination

f. to stop something bad from affecting you for a period of time; to delay something

g. beginning to exist or is happening now

h. a set of actions that is the official or accepted way of doing something

i. to be closely related to or linked; cannot be considered separately from each other

j. a medicine or a set of drugs used to treat an illness or improve a physical condition

♀ Vocabulary Practice

Complete the following sentences with the words shown in the box. Change the grammatical form if necessary.

1. The disease can be cured if treatment is started as soon as it is (   ).

2. Having regular exercise can help you look younger, feel better and (   ) illness.

3. The doctor gave me a prescription for some pain (   ) and

told me to stay in bed as much as possible for a week.

4. In order to find a method to treat the disease, a number of research projects are currently (   ).

5. I will go through the (   ) with you step by step to check if there is any problem.

6. The company claims that these are truly organic products which contain no (   ) chemicals.

7. She held her hands above her eyes to (   ) them from the strong sunlight.

8. The cyclist (   ) emergency surgery yesterday after a collision with a car.

9. Having problems with short-term memory and thinking skills is one of the main symptoms of (   ).

10. A hospital chef's menu should (   ) with a nutritionist's advice when preparing meals for diabetic patients.

✍ Comprehension

Read the following sentences on the content of the article and choose the best answer.

1. What is expected to happen to the number of people who have dementia by 2050?
     a. They will be treated using a combination of new drugs.
     b. There will be three times as many of them.
     c. The popularity of dementia will decline and go out of fashion.
     d. Some will become more seriously ill and others will get better.

2. The article says that Alzheimer's disease is one of the . . .
     a. diseases that all old people suffer from.
     b. normal effects of living for a long time in a city.
     c. most common types of dementia.
     d. least dangerous forms of mental illness.

3. What problem does the blood-brain barrier cause?
     a. It makes it hard to treat neurodegenerative diseases.
     b. It carries signals from one side of the brain to the other.

c. It is the location in the brain where Alzheimer's starts.

d. It opens and causes pain when old people try to think.

4. What do researchers believe is connected with a loss of memory and cognition in Alzheimer's sufferers?

   a. fewer valuable experiences in life or a continuous feeling of boredom

   b. a poor diet in later years, when the brain needs more nourishment

   c. smoking at a young age, before the brain can fully develop

   d. a higher deposition of amyloid in that area of the brain

5. How did David and Kim Shorr feel about joining the clinical trial?

   a. They knew about the trial very well because it was explained on TV.

   b. They were afraid to join it because David's Alzheimer's was not serious.

   c. They agreed to join it even though they didn't know what the trial was.

   d. They laughed and thought it was a joke when they got a letter about it.

ⓘ Coffee Break

Beta-amyloid and the Amyloid Hypothesis

In Alzheimer's disease, brain cells that process, store and retrieve information degenerate and die. Although scientists do not yet know the underlying cause of this destruction, they have identified several possible culprits.

One prime suspect is a microscopic brain protein fragment called beta-amyloid, a sticky compound that accumulates in the brain, disrupting communication between brain cells and eventually killing them. Some researchers believe that flaws in the processes governing production, accumulation or disposal of beta-amyloid are the primary cause of Alzheimer's. This theory is called "the amyloid hypothesis."

Source: *Alzheimer's Association* Updated in March 2017 https://www.alz.org/

📚 Words & Phrases

retrieve: 〜を取り戻す
culprit: （問題の）原因、発端
microscopic: 微細な
compound: 複合物
flaw: 不具合、欠陥
govern: 〜を制御する、支配する
the Amyloid Hypothesis:
《医》アミロイド仮説

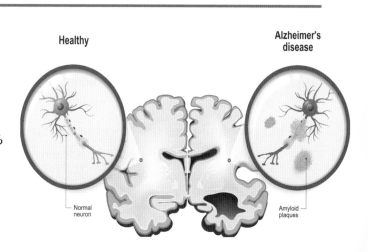

Healthy

Alzheimer's disease

Normal neuron

Amyloid plaques

Unit 9

Link Between Diet and Brain

⌘Pre-reading⌘

1970年代の初頭にファーストフードが日本に上陸して以来、「安さ」と「速さ」を売り物にする様々な外食産業が繁栄し、人々の食生活にまつわる環境が大いに変化して来ました。栄養のバランスが取れていない、高カロリーな食べ物の過剰摂取は、肥満や糖尿病などの健康問題の一因であることはすでに広く理解されています。オーストラリア国立大学による最新の研究によって、長期にわたる不健康な食生活及び運動不足が、実は私たちの脳機能に障害をもたらす可能性のあることが明らかになりました。

⌘Reading⌘

The average person worldwide has added the equivalent of a burger, fries and soft drink in calories to their daily diet in the last 50 years, a trend that researchers have found is eating away at the brain.

An Australian National University study has found a link between irreversible declines in brain function and unhealthy lifestyles that start as 5 soon as early childhood.

The link between rapid brain degeneration and type-2 diabetes is well-known already.

New research led by ANU professor Nicolas Cherbuin has discovered strong evidence that unhealthy eating habits and lack of exercise for long 10 periods of time also put people at serious risk of developing dementia and brain shrinkage.

The research reports about 30 percent of the world's adult population is either overweight or obese, and more than 10 percent of all adults will suffer from type-2 diabetes by 2030. 15

Professor Cherbuin said fast food diets and little to no exercise were permanently reducing brain function.

"What has become really apparent in our investigation is that advice for people to reduce their risk of brain problems, including their risk of getting dementia, is most commonly given in their 60s or later, when the 20 'timely prevention' horse has already bolted," he said.

"Unless we do something about it early, we accumulate this risk, and when the disease becomes detectable then much of the damage is done," he said.

"The damage done is pretty much irreversible once a person reaches 25 midlife, so we urge everyone to eat healthy and get in shape as early as possible, preferably in childhood but certainly by early adulthood."

The research, published in the journal *Frontiers in Neuroendocrinology*, found results of an ACT-based study on brain health shared common patterns with more than 200 international studies. 30

Professor Cherbuin said it showed Australia was not isolated from the health problems posed by obesity, despite popular thinking that the issue was worse in other countries such as the United States.

His team's message isn't intended to blame people for their health decisions. Solutions aren't simple and won't be found only by telling people 35 to look after themselves better, Professor Cherbuin said.

The causes of the problem include the environment obese and overweight people live in, which makes it harder to make healthy choices. Cheap and widely available fast food, and unclear dietary information on packaging, are some barriers to making better lifestyle decisions. 40

"We should develop a social and economic environment, and also an education environment, that give us the tools to live more healthy lives," Professor Cherbuin said.

🐚 Words & Phrases

[l. 3] **eat away at ～:** （どんどん食べて）徐々に～を蝕む
[l. 4] **Australian National University:** オーストラリア国立大学。首都キャンベラ
        にあるオーストラリア唯一の国立大学
[l. 16] **little to no:** 皆無かそれに近い
[l. 21] **horse has already bolted:** すでに手遅れである　cf. to close the stable
        door after the horse has bolted: 馬が逃げてから馬小屋の扉を閉める (慣用
        表現：悪い事態が起きてから対策を立てること)
[l. 28] **Frontiers in Neuroendocrinology:** 1980 年に創刊された神経内分泌学に関
        する季刊の学術雑誌
[l. 29] **ACT-based study:** オーストラリア首都特別地域研究 (ACT=the Australia
        Capital Territory)
[l. 32] **pose:** ～をもたらす

☑Vocabulary Check

Match each word in the box with the most appropriate definition shown below.

Words	Definitions	Words	Definitions
equivalent		accumulate	
irreversible		preferably	
degeneration		intend	
shrinkage		blame	
permanently		dietary	

Definitions:

a. a reduction in the size of something or the process of getting smaller

b. impossible to change or return to a previous condition

c. to say or think that someone did something wrong or is responsible for something bad happening

d. in an ideal way; wanted more

e. having the same amount, value, purpose, qualities and etc.

f. to collect or increase an amount of something gradually over a period of time

g. relating to the food and drink a person is usually having

h. the process by which something gets worse

i. in a way that continues without changing or ending

j. to have in mind as a purpose or goal

⚲ Vocabulary Practice

Complete the following sentences with the words shown in the box. Change the grammatical form if necessary.

1. Once you have received this vaccine, you will be (　　　　　) immune from getting infected by the virus again.

2. This product is not (　　　　　) to treat, cure or prevent any heart disease.

3. It's not easy to lose weight because (　　　　　) habits can be very difficult to change.

4. She is doing a/an (　　　　　) job in the new hospital but for a higher salary.

5. The newly developed treatment caused almost a 50 percent (   ) in tumor size for most patients.

6. Take this tablet only once a day, (   ) before you go to bed.

7. Smoking cigarettes for many years has brought (   ) damage to his lungs.

8. High blood pressure can cause (   ) of heart muscles.

9. Cholesterol, calcium and other substances (   ) on the walls of arteries.

10. Two people were injured, and the speeding driver was (   ) for the car accident.

✎ Comprehension

Choose the correct phrase to complete the sentence in line with the article.

1. A study has found a link between irreversible (   ) and unhealthy lifestyles that start as soon as early childhood.

    a. methods used in education

    b. decay happening near the spine

    c. reductions in brain activity

    d. improvements in society

2. The research reports about 30 percent of the world's (   ) over-weight or obese.

    a. people over 18 years old are

    b. teachers are planning to become

    c. children resist being called

    d. pets don't mind looking

3. Unless we do something about our diet early, we accumulate risk, and when the disease becomes detectable then (   ).

    a. it is too late to regain good health

    b. we don't mind the way it has developed

    c. doctors can solve the problem

    d. most people give up trying

4. Australia was not isolated from the health problems posed by obesity, (   ) the issue was worse in other countries.

   a. but the overall extent of
   b. even though many people believed
   c. because top experts thought
   d. and they worked to prove

5. Cheap and widely available fast food, and unclear dietary information on packaging, are (   ) better lifestyle decisions.

   a. preventing people from adopting
   b. beneficial for helping people get
   c. useful options when considering
   d. terrible ways to teach about

ⓘ Coffee Break

How many calories should I eat a day?

When most of us think of calories, we think of how fattening a food is. In dietary terms, calories are the amount of energy that a food provides. The definition of a calorie is the amount of energy needed to raise the temperature of 1 gram (g) of water 1° Celsius.

Around 20 percent of the energy we take in is used for brain metabolism. Most of the rest is used in basal metabolism, the energy we need when in a resting state, for functions such as blood circulation, digestion, and breathing. We also need mechanical energy for our skeletal muscles, to maintain posture and move around.

According to the 2015-2020 Dietary Guidelines for Americans, women are likely to need between 1,600 and 2,400 calories a day, and men from 2,000 to 3,000. However, this depends on their age, size, height, lifestyle, overall health, and activity level.

Source: https://www.medicalnewstoday.com/articles

☕ Words & Phrases

term: 言い方
brain metabolism: 脳代謝
basal metabolism: 基礎代謝
mechanical energy:
力学的エネルギー
skeletal muscle: 骨格筋

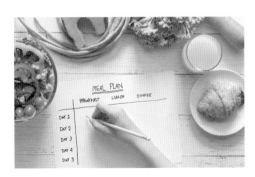

☺ Useful Expressions 3

Medical Examination, Pains and Symptoms

Doctor: Good afternoon, Ms. Adams. How are you feeling today?

Patient: Well, about two days ago I started feeling

rather tired.
quite weary.
kind of sluggish.
a bit feverish.
really nauseous.

Doctor: Oh, that's too bad. Do you have any other symptoms?

Patient: Yes, actually, yesterday afternoon, I

started having heart palpitations.
noticed this rash on my legs.
felt a sharp pain in my abdomen.
began throwing up.
had intense stiffness in my joints.
heard a loud ringing in my ears.

Doctor: How long did that continue?

Patient: It lasted until this morning. That's why I made my appointment last night.

Doctor: Well, let me ask you some more questions. Have you been under much stress lately?

Patient: Yes, I have. My job has been very busy.

Doctor: Have you had any change in your diet or appetite?

Patient: No, nothing really.

Doctor: Have you had any

cramps?
fainting spells?
trouble breathing?
lost of memory?
mood swings?
constipation?

Patient: Well, yes. I have.

Doctor: Well, I would like to | run a few tests.
do a blood test.
get a CT scan.
take an x-ray.

Patient: Can we do it today, or will I need to make another appointment?

Doctor: We can do the test today, but I'm sorry, you'll need to come back for the results.

🔖 Words & Phrases

weary:（肉体的に、精神的に）疲れた

sluggish: のろのろした、活気のない

feverish: 熱っぽい　☞ -ish（接尾辞）: 〜の性質をもつ、〜ような、〜っぽい、〜気味の

nauseous: むかむかするような、吐き気がする　cf. nausea: 吐き気

heart palpitation: 心臓の動悸

rash: 発疹、ふきでもの

a sharp pain: 鋭い痛み　cf. a dull pain: 鈍い痛み

to throw up: 〜を嘔吐する

stiffness:（筋肉の）凝り

ringing in one's ears:（両耳で起きる）耳鳴り　cf. ringing in one's ear:（片耳で起きる）耳鳴り

diet: 食事、食生活

appetite: 食欲

cramps: 激しい腹痛、生理痛、（手足の）けいれん

fainting spells: 失神の発作

mood swing: 感情の起伏

constipation: 便秘　☞ be constipated の形がよく使われる。(例)I have been constipated for a week.

CT scan: CT 検査、computed tomographic scan

Unit 10

Vaping Boom among Teens

⌘Pre-reading⌘

　近年日本でも、火を使わずに喫煙できる電子たばこの使用が急速に拡大しています。様々な種類のものが存在しますが、例えば、フィリップ・モリス社製のIQOS（アイコス）は、ペースト状に加工されたタバコの葉が入っているヒートスティックを加熱することで、蒸気を発生させ、ニコチンやその他の成分を吸引する喫煙具です。世界保健機関（WHO）は、電子たばこは健康に有害であると指摘しています。最近、アメリカの高校生の間で電子たばこの使用が著しく増えています。

⌘Reading⌘

Twice as many high school students used nicotine-tinged electronic cigarettes in 2018 compared with the previous year, an unprecedented jump found in a large annual survey of teen smoking, drinking and drug use.

It was the largest single-year increase in the survey's 44-year history, far surpassing a mid-1970s surge in marijuana smoking. 5

The findings echo those of a government survey earlier this year. That survey also found a dramatic rise in vaping among children and prompted federal regulators to press for new restriction measures.

Experts attribute the jump to newer versions of e-cigarettes, like those by Juul Labs Inc. that resemble computer flash drives and can be used dis- 10 creetly.

Trina Hale, a junior at South Charleston High School in West Virginia, said vaping — specifically Juul — exploded at her school this year.

"They can put it in their sleeve or their pocket. They can do it wherever, whenever. They can do it in class if they're sneaky about it," she said. 15

Olivia Turman, a high school freshman, said she too has seen kids "hit their vape in class."

The federally funded survey is conducted by University of Michigan researchers and has been operating since 1975. This year's findings are based on responses from about 45,000 students in grades 8, 10 and 12 in schools 20 across the country. It found 1 in 5 high school seniors reported having vaped nicotine in the previous month.

After vaping and alcohol, the most common thing teens use is mari-

juana, the survey found. About 1 in 4 students said they had used marijuana at least once in the past year. It was more common in older kids — 25
about 1 in 17 high school seniors said they use marijuana every day.

Overall, marijuana smoking is about the same level as it was the past
few years. Vaping of marijuana rose, however.

More teens, however, are saying no to lots of other substances. Usage
of alcohol, cigarettes, cocaine, LSD, ecstasy, heroin and opioid pills all de- 30
clined.

Experts say it's not clear what's behind those trends, especially since
the nation is in the midst of the deadliest drug overdose epidemic ever.

One leading theory is that kids today are staying home and communi-
cating on smartphones rather than hanging out and smoking, drinking or 35
trying drugs.

Drug experimentation is a group activity. What about vaping? "Vaping
mostly is an individual activity," said David Jernigan, a Boston University
researcher who tracks alcohol use.

The vaping explosion is a big worry, however. Health officials say nico- 40
tine is harmful to developing brains. Some researchers also believe vaping
will make kids more likely to take up cigarettes, and perhaps later try other
drugs.

🐚 Words & Phrases

[l. 1]　**nicotine-tinged:** ニコチンを含む〜
[l. 5]　**surge:** 急増
[l. 6]　**echo:** 〜を反映する
[l. 7]　**prompt A to 〜:** A に〜するように促す
[l. 8]　**press for:** 〜を強く求める
[l. 9]　**attribute A to B:** A の原因を B のせいにする
[l. 10]　**Juul Labs Inc:** カリフォルニア州に拠点を置く電子タバコのメーカー。2018 年
　　　　　9 月の時点でアメリカ国内の電子タバコ市場の約 70％のシェアを持つ。
[l. 18]　**federally funded survey:** 連邦政府資金による調査
[l. 33]　**in the midst of:** 〜の真っただ中で

☑Vocabulary Check

Match each word in the box with the most appropriate definition shown below.

Words	Definitions	Words	Definitions
unprecedented		discreetly	
surpass		substance	
vape		overdose	
restriction		epidemic	
resemble		track	

Definitions:

a. never having happened or existed in the past

b. too much of a drug taken or given at one time, either intentionally or by accident

c. to look like or to be similar to someone or something

d. to be better or bigger than something else or to go beyond what was expected

e. a drug that people can get addicted to, especially an illegal drug

f. to breathe the vapor produced by an electronic cigarette into your lungs

g. in a way that is careful not to attract too much attention or by keeping something secret

h. an official limit or control on what people are allowed to do

i. to find out more about something by following its movement or development over a period of time

j. a particular problem that seriously affects a lot of people at the same time

♀ Vocabulary Practice

Complete the following sentences with the words shown in the box. Change the grammatical form if necessary.

1. The virus' level of infection became a/an (   ) and led to more poverty and crime in the country.

2. The increase in (   ) by kids and young people is a serious public health threat.

3. She came in late and found a place to sit as (   ) as possible

because the teacher had already started his lecture.

4. According to the *New York Times*, the US Department of Defense has released videos of UFOs, which is (   ) in history.

5. In spite of having a great talent in music, he died from a massive (   ) of heroin.

6. My twin sisters (   ) each other more strongly when they were younger.

7. The study (   ) the careers of 1,500 doctors who trained at the national medical school.

8. In the end, the number of people who were infected by coronavirus (   ) the number that the government had predicted.

9. Chinese officials called on America to ease (   ) preventing the export of high-tech goods to China.

10. Cocaine is a harmful and addictive (   ) which is made from the leaves of the coca plant.

✍ Comprehension

Underline the words in each sentence that don't match the content of the article and correct them.

1. The number of teens using nicotine-tinged electronic cigarettes largely increased in the 1990s, far surpassing a mid-1970s surge in marijuana smoking.
   ⇒ (   )

2. Experts attribute the jump to newer versions of e-cigarettes that are cheaper to buy and can be used discreetly.
   ⇒ (   )

3. This year's findings are examining the habits of over 45,000 students in grades 8, 10 and 12 in schools across the country.
   ⇒ (   )

4. More teens, however, are interested in trying many other substances.
   ⇒ (   )

5. Health officials say nicotine stimulates young peoples' brains.
   ⇒ (   )

ⓘ Coffee Break

Are e-cigarette and other vaping products dangerous?

E-cigarette emissions typically contain nicotine and other toxic substances that are harmful to both users and non-users who are exposed to the aerosols secondhand. Some products claiming to be nicotine-free have been found to contain nicotine.

Evidence reveals that these products are harmful to health and are not safe. However, it is too early to provide a clear answer on the long-term impact of using them or being exposed to them.

They are particularly risky when used by children and adolescents. Nicotine is highly addictive and young people's brains develop up to their mid-twenties. Exposure to nicotine for children and adolescents can have long-lasting, damaging effects on brain development and there is risk of nicotine addiction.

Source: https://www.who.int/news-room

🕮 Words & Phrases ─────────────────────────

emission: 排出物
aerosol: エアロゾル（噴霧物）
adolescent: 青年期の若者

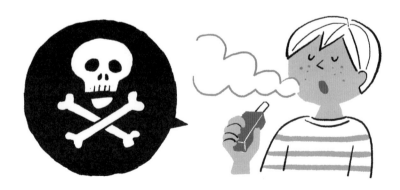

Unit 11

Vehicle for Drug Delivery

⌘Pre-reading⌘

　ナノ粒子（超微粒子）は、一般的な粒子と違い、その小ささゆえの特別な性質を持っています。ナノ粒子とは、通常100nm以下の粒子を指す場合が多いです。最新の医療への応用研究では、金ナノ粒子は免疫系のB細胞（骨髄由来の細胞）の機能に干渉せず、しかもワクチンや薬の効き目を最大限に発揮できる安全なツールとして利用できることがわかりました。それは、なぜなのでしょうか。金ナノ粒子の潜在的可能性を見ていきましょう。

⌘Reading⌘

52　Gold nanoparticles could be a safe tool for improving the effectiveness of vaccines and other medicines that need to target the B cells of the immune system, according to new research.

　The number of medical uses for nanoparticles has grown steadily over the last 20 years. The human body tolerates gold well, and the metal is easy ⁵ to manipulate. In the form of nanoparticles, gold offers the potential to target cells in specific ways. Drug delivery in precision medicine could be a promising area.

53　Previous studies have already established that gold nanoparticles can work with larger immune cells, such as macrophages, in safe ways. 10

　Now, for the first time, scientists have investigated how gold nanoparticles interact with B lymphocytes, or white blood cells, which are smaller and less easy to manage.

　B cells are largely responsible for the production of antibodies in the immune system. 15

　"Nanoparticles," says co-senior study author Carole Bourquin, a professor in the faculties of medicine and science at the University of Geneva in Switzerland, "can form a protective vehicle for vaccines — or other drugs — to specifically deliver them where they can be most effective while sparing other cells." 20

54 Effect of gold nanoparticles on B cells

　Bourquin and her colleagues investigated interactions between different forms of gold nanoparticles and "freshly isolated human B lymphocytes."

　They found that the type of surface on the gold nanoparticles and their shape had a significant effect on their interactions with B cells. 25

Uncoated spherical gold nanoparticles proved unsuitable because they showed a tendency to form clumps.

The best performers were the polymer-coated, spherical gold nanoparticles. These were stable and did not interfere with the function of the B cells.

Rod-shaped gold nanoparticles, on the other hand, were not usable because they reduced the immune response rather than activating it. The researchers suggest that this could be because they were heavier and likely interfered with processes in the cell membranes. 30

Potential of gold 'nanodrugs'

To be effective, vaccine drugs need to reach B cells before the body destroys them. Using gold nanoparticles to deliver them could be an effective way to preserve the drugs during their perilous journey to their targets. 35

B cells can be targets not only for vaccines but also for drugs that treat other diseases, such as cancer and autoimmune conditions.

The researchers see the gold nanoparticles that they have developed 40 as a potential vehicle for delivering drugs directly to B cells.

Such a delivery vehicle could reduce the dosage of drugs and their associated side effects.

🐚 Words & Phrases ━━━━━━━━━━━━━━━━━━━━━━━━━━━

[l. 2] **B cell:** B 細胞。脊椎動物の免疫系における白血球のサブタイプの一つであるリンパ球の一種

[l. 7] **precision medicine:** プレシジョン・メディシン（精密医療）。患者の個人レベルで細胞の遺伝子分析を行い、最適な投薬及び治療方法を施す医療

[l. 10] **macrophage:** マクロファージ。白血球の一種で、免疫機能の中心的役割を担うアメーバ状の大形細胞

[l. 12] **B lymphocyte:** B リンパ球（ B cell）

[l. 14] **antibody:** 抗体 (cf. antigen 抗原)

[l. 17] **University of Geneva:** ジュネーブ大学、1559 年に創設されたスイスのジュネーブにある大学

[l. 19] **spare:** 〜に危害を加えない

[l. 28] **polymer-coated:** 高分子化合物によって被覆された、ポロマー加工の

[l. 30] **rod-shaped:** 棒状の

[l. 33] **process:** 突起。組織の主要構造部から飛び出ている部分

[l. 33] **cell membrane:** 細胞膜

[l. 37] **perilous:** 危険な

[l. 39] **autoimmune:** 自己免疫の

☑Vocabulary Check

Match each word in the box with the most appropriate definition shown below.

Words	Definitions	Words	Definitions
immune		colleague	
tolerate		surface	
manipulate		tendency	
potential		vaccine	
vehicle		interfere with	

Definitions:

a. a means of carrying or transporting something
b. someone you work with in a company or organization
c. to control someone or something in a skillful manner
d. a general response or development in a particular and predictable direction
e. resistant to or unaffected by something harmful, especially a bacteria or disease
f. to allow something to exist or take place without trying to stop it
g. to prevent something from working effectively or to stop it from happening
h. the outside or top layer of something
i. having or showing the capacity to develop into something in the future
j. a substance containing a weak form of a virus or bacteria, given to a person or animal to provide protection against that disease

♀ Vocabulary Practice

Complete the following sentences with the words shown in the box. Change the grammatical form if necessary.

1. It is said that coronavirus can survive on the (   ) of plastic or steel for up to 72 hours.

2. A medical method developed a decade ago has the (   ) to cure the new disease.

3. His (   ) became worried about whether or not he was ill, since he was absent from work without notifying them.

4. This medical device is designed so that it is easy for a doctor to (   ) during surgery.

5. Frequent arguing by parents may (   ) a child's performance at school.

6. If your (   ) system is damaged, a cold which normally takes a few days to clear up can take several weeks.

7. Coronavirus is spreading around the world, and people are waiting for the development of an effective (   ) that can protect against it.

8. We can't (   ) smoking in the hospital because it is bad for health.

9. Patients suffering from this disease have a/an (   ) to lose weight in a short period of time.

10. The police officer asked the driver whether he was the registered owner of the (   ).

✍ Comprehension

Read the following sentences on the content of the article and choose the best answer.

1. For how many years has the number of medical uses for nanoparticles steadily grown?

   a. The uses have grown in recent years.
   b. The uses have grown for over the last 20 years.
   c. The uses have grown during the last few years.
   d. The uses have grown for less than 15 years.

2. What kind of cells have previous studies already established that gold nanoparticles can work with?

   a. Gold nanoparticles can cautiously interact with stem cells.
   b. Gold nanoparticles can toxically interact with smaller sleeper cells.
   c. Gold nanoparticles can passively interact with mutating cancer cells.
   d. Gold nanoparticles can safely interact with larger immune cells.

3. Because nanoparticles can form a protective vehicle for some drugs, what benefit do they offer?

   a. They keep the body safe from side effects that can damage the immune system.
   b. They can deliver drugs to the most effective locations while affecting other cells less.
   c. They often speed up the recovery time for patients with allergic reactions.
   d. They are a less expensive form of treatment because less drugs are needed.

4. What two characteristics of gold nanoparticles significantly effect their interactions with B cells?

   a. the structural form of the gold nanoparticles and their color
   b. the source of the material used in making the gold nanoparticles and their cost
   c. the curvature of the gold nanoparticles' base and their age
   d. the type of surface on the gold nanoparticles and their shape

5. What regularly prevents vaccine drugs from being effective?

   a. The drugs cluster in the liver and lose their potency.
   b. The gold nanoparticles decrease in number over time.
   c. The body destroys the drugs before they can reach B cells.
   d. The disease grows too quickly for the dosage prescribed.

ⓘ Coffee Break

How small is a nanoparticle?

It is hard to grasp just how small a nanoparticle is. So, imagine if a nanoparticle was the size of a football. This image shows how atoms, cells and organisms would compare at a more familiar scale.

Source: https//: www.sciencelearn.org.nz/

🍃 Words & Phrases ────────────────────

compare: ～に匹敵する

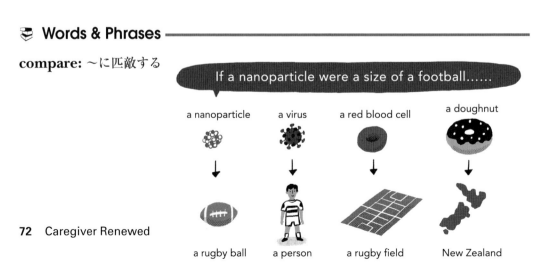

If a nanoparticle were a size of a football……

| a nanoparticle | a virus | a red blood cell | a doughnut |
| a rugby ball | a person | a rugby field | New Zealand |

Unit 12

Multimorbidity vs. Quality of Life

⌘Pre-reading⌘

　年齢を重ねると、高血圧、糖尿病や慢性心不全など、複数の慢性疾患を抱える人口の割合が増えていきます。このようにいくつかの健康問題が併存しているために、中心となる疾患に焦点を当て難い状態を、マルチモビディティ(multimorbidity＝多疾患併存状態)と呼び、近年特に高齢者医療の分野で注目されてきている考え方です。複数の慢性疾患を患っていると、私たちは身体的な困難に直面するだけでなく、精神面及びその延長上にある QOL（quality of life）においても影響を受けるのです。

⌘Reading⌘

57 　After studying thousands of people for over a decade, researchers have concluded that living with multiple chronic conditions can seriously affect a person's brain health and mental well-being, speeding up forms of memory loss and increasing the risk of suicide.

　Recent research has shown that people living with a chronic condition 5 may report a decrease in their quality of life.

　Quality of life refers to a person's level of physical, psychological, and social functioning, among other features.

58 　However, as the World Health Organization (WHO) notes, "People living with a long term condition often have multiple rather than a single 10 condition." This is called "multimorbidity," and according to the WHO, it is very "common and has been rising in prevalence over recent years." For instance, one study in a Scottish population found that 42.2% of participants of all ages had one or more chronic conditions, and that 23.2% of the study population had multimorbidity. 15

　It may come as no surprise that living with multiple chronic conditions can take its toll on a person's general well-being. However, a large new longitudinal study now confirms that multimorbidity does not just affect physical health; it can also severely impact mental health and hasten cognitive decline. 20

59 　The research team, which Dr. Melissa Wei led, also came up with a new test: a multimorbidity weighted index (MWI), which allows them to predict how different coexisting conditions interact and to what degree these in-

74　Caregiver Renewed

teractions may impact a person's quality of life — particularly their cognitive health. 25

Dr. Wei and colleagues calculated the MWI of 14,265 participants — of whom 60% were female — who contributed 73,700 interviews. The mean age of the participants at baseline was 67.

The researchers followed the participants over a period of 14 years, and they assessed for various changes in their cognitive abilities, including epi- 30 sodic and working memory. These forms of memory allow people to make day-to-day decisions based on momentary contexts and factors.

The researchers found that those with high MWI scores were at risk of cognitive decline. In fact, the higher they scored, the faster their cognitive abilities — such as word recall and simple math calculations — appeared 35 to decline over the 14-year study period.

These results follow another set of alarming findings that Dr. Wei and her team published last year — in *The Journal of the American Geriatric Society* — which showed that people with high MWI scores had more than twice the risk of dying by suicide than those with lower MWI scores. 40

Participants with high MWI scores were also more likely to have poorer mental health overall. For that study, the researchers looked at data from 252,002 participants.

📖 Words & Phrases

[l. 3]   **forms of:** 様々な形の
[l. 8]   **social functioning:** 社会的機能
[l. 16]   **come as no surprise:** なんら驚く事ではない
[l. 17]   **take a toll on～:** ～を損ねる
[l. 30]   **episodic memory:** エピソード記憶
[l. 31]   **working memory:** 作業記憶
[l. 32]   **day-to-day:** 日常的な
[l. 38]   **The Journal of the American Geriatric Society:** アメリカ老年医学会ジャ
          ーナル

☑Vocabulary Check

Match each word in the box with the most appropriate definition shown below.

Words	Definitions	Words	Definitions
chronic		hasten	
well-being		cognitive	
morbidity		decline	
participant		mean	
longitudinal		alarming	

Definitions:

a. relating to conscious intellectual activity such as thinking, reasoning or understanding

b. occupying a middle or intermediate position between two extremes

c. the state of feeling healthy and happy

d. continuing for a long time, especially a disease or something bad

e. examined or done over a long period of time

f. causing people to feel in danger or to be suddenly worried or frightened

g. to make something happen sooner or more quickly

h. a person who takes part in or is involved in a particular activity

i. to gradually become less, worse or lower

j. a word used to describe how often a disease occurs in a specific area or how many people have it in a particular population

♀ Vocabulary Practice

Complete the following sentences with the words shown in the box. Change the grammatical form if necessary.

1. They found a/an ( ) number of people who were infected by coronavirus.

2. ( ) in this experiment are asked to report what they eat and drink for a week.

3. Profits have ( ) as a result of the recent drop in sales due to the pandemic situation facing the nation.

4. There is no doubt that poor medical equipment and sub-standard treat-

ment (   ) his death.

5. As she suffers from quite severe (   ) liver disease, she is willing to try any new medicine available.

6. The doctor found that some (   ) functions in his brain became impaired after the car accident.

7. Risk-taking behavior is one of the major causes of (   ) and mortality among young people.

8. The (   ) age of a group of three people aged 10, 13, and 22 is 15.

9. After a/an (   ) study, researchers were finally able to characterize all the symptoms that this disease might cause.

10. The old couple become cheerful and have a sense of (   ) whenever they see their grandchildren.

✍ Comprehension

Choose the correct phrase to complete the sentence in line with the article.

1. Quality of life refers to (   ), psychological, and social functioning, among other features.
    a. a way to measure job
    b. problems in personal
    c. success in mental
    d. someone's amount of physical

2. It may come as no surprise that (   ) conditions can take its toll on a person's general well-being.
    a. having several ongoing health
    b. thinking about complicated
    c. struggling against social
    d. a change in employment

3. Episodic memory and working memory allow people to (   ) based on momentary contexts and factors.
    a. choose what to do in everyday situations
    b. improve their situation
    c. change dangerous pressure
    d. determine the best opinion

4. The (   ), the faster their cognitive abilities appeared to decline over the 14-year study period.

    a. slower they moved

    b. sicker they felt

    c. higher their MWI score

    d. more they smoked

5. For the study in the article, the researchers (   ) 252,002 participants.

    a. measured the heart rates of

    b. examined results collected on

    c. conducted interviews with

    d. developed questions for

ⓘ Coffee Break

What is Quality of Life?

WHO defines Quality of Life as an individual's perception of their position in life in the context of the culture and value systems in which they live and in relation to their goals, expectations, standards and concerns. It is a broad ranging concept affected in a complex way by the person's physical health, psychological state, personal beliefs, social relationships and their relationship to salient features of their environment.

Source: https://www.who.int/healthinfo/survey/whogol-qualityoflife/en/

⮻ Words & Phrases

perception: 認識、感じ方
salient: 目立った、顕著な

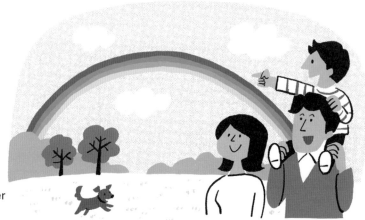

☺ Useful Expressions 4

Pandemic Telephone Diagnosis

Diagnosis Nurse: You've reached the Pandemic Hotline.

Caller: Hello, I am afraid I might have COVID-19. How can I get tested?

Diagnosis Nurse: Before we can test you, we need to check your symptoms. Can I ask you some questions to diagnose your condition?

Caller: Sure.

Diagnosis Nurse: Do you currently have a fever?

Caller: Yes, I do. I've had a fever for three days.

Diagnosis Nurse: What is your temperature?

Caller: It is now 37.8 degrees Celsius.

Diagnosis Nurse: What other symptoms do you have? And, how long have you had them?

Caller: I have had

a headache	for five days.
a stomachache	for one week.
vomiting	since last night.
body aches	since yesterday morning.
no sense of taste	off and on.
a strong cough	since this afternoon.
dizziness	all day long.

Diagnosis Nurse: Those symptoms

| don't suggest you have COVID-19. |
| suggest you might have COVID-19. |

Please see your doctor.

Caller: Oh, I see.

Diagnosis Nurse: So, please contact [XXX-XXXX] for instructions about getting tested.

Caller: Okay. Thank you for your help.

🐟 Words & Phrases

diagnose: 診断する
vomiting: 嘔吐　cf. to vomit: 嘔吐する
a sense of taste or smell: 味覚や臭覚
off and on: 断続的に
degree Celsius: 摂氏温度（℃）　cf. degree Fahrenheit: 華氏温度（℉）

摂氏/華氏換算式：　$℃ × 1.8 + 32 = ℉$

	Celsius ℃	Fahrenheit ℉
氷の融点	0 ℃	32 ℉
人の平熱	36 ℃	96.8 ℉
水の沸点	100 ℃	212 ℉
太陽の表面温度	6000 ℃	10832 ℉

⛬ Let's check !

How many words and phrases do you know?

pandemic
epidemic
outbreak
herd immunity
infection cluster
transmission
community spread
person-to-person contact
respiratory droplet
infectious pathogens
preventative measures
social distancing
quarantine
hand sanitizer, surface disinfectant
first responder

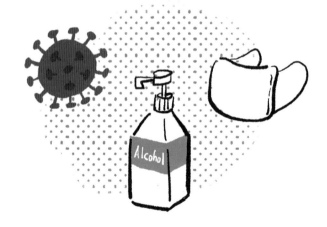

Unit 13

Save the Planet Diet

⌘Pre-reading⌘

ロンドンに集まった科学者たちが人間や地球にやさしい食事を提案しています。それはどのようなものでしょう。地球と人間は別々の存在ではなく、相互依存の関係にあることを強調するプラネタリーヘルス（planetary health）という観点から考えると、私達の食生活が地球環境にやさしいかどうかを詳しく見ていきましょう。

⌘Reading⌘

62　Scientists in London say they have found the best diet for both humans and the planet.

If the world followed the so-called "planetary health" diet, the scientists told Reuters, each year more than 11 million early deaths could be prevented.　5

For the health of the planet, they claim the same diet would reduce greenhouse gases and save more land, water and animals.

This new food plan is the result of a three-year project organized by The Lancet health journal. It involved 37 experts from 16 countries.

63　Tim Lang, a professor at Britain's University of London, co-led the re-　10 search. He told Reuters, "The food we eat and how we produce it determine the health of people and the planet, and we are currently getting this seriously wrong."

Lang added that the world's population is expected to grow to 10 billion people by 2050. If we want to feed everyone, he explained, we all need　15 to change what we eat and the way we eat by "improving food production and reducing food waste."

64　So, what do you eat on the planetary health diet?

The scientists who created this diet say it is largely plant-based but still has small amounts of dairy, fish and meat. The diet calls for cutting red　20 meat and sugar by 50 percent and doubling the amount of nuts, fruits, vegetables and legumes.

65　Food situations around the world are not equal. In certain areas, this would mean great changes. People in North America, for example, eat 6.5

times the recommended amount of red meat. On the other hand, people 25
in South Asia eat only half the amount suggested by the new planetary
health diet.

Meeting the targets for vegetables would need big changes in other
areas. In sub-Saharan Africa, people on average eat 7.5 times the suggested
amount of vegetables like potatoes and cassava. 30

Walter Willet of Harvard University in the United States also talked to
Reuters about the planetary health diet. He said that more than 800 million people around the world do not get enough food while many more
have very unhealthy diets.

The scientists admit their goal will be difficult to achieve. But for them 35
doing nothing is also not an option. Willet said, "If we can't quite make it,
it's better to try and get as close as we can."

Words & Phrases

[l. 4] **Reuters:** ロイター。国際ニュース通信社
[l. 9] **The Lancet:** ランセット週刊医学雑誌。世界で最も読まれている医学雑誌の一つ
[l. 10] **Britain's University of London:** ロンドン大学。1836年に創立されたイギリ
スのカレッジ制の連合大学
[l. 22] **legume:** マメ科植物
[l. 30] **cassava:** キャッサバ。イモノキ属の熱帯低木、ユカとも呼ばれる
[l. 31] **Harvard University:** アメリカ合衆国マサチューセッツ州ボストン近郊ケン
ブリッジに位置する総合私立大学。1636年に設立されたアメリカ最古の大学

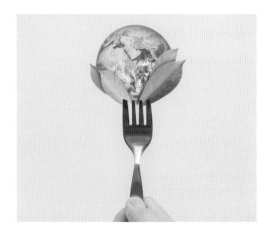

☑Vocabulary Check

Match each word in the box with the most appropriate definition shown below.

Words	Definitions	Words	Definitions
diet		feed	
planetary		dairy	
prevent		suggest	
claim		admit	
determine		achieve	

Definitions:

a. food that people regularly eat
b. reach by effort
c. provide with food
d. assert, insist
e. ensure that something does not happen
f. relating to the earth
g. agree that it is true
h. food made from milk
i. put forward for consideration
j. firmly decide

♀ Vocabulary Practice

Complete the following sentences with the words shown in the box. Change the grammatical form if necessary.

1. It is always our father who (   ) the destination of our vacation trip.

2. Doctors (   ) that we do some exercise regularly.

3. The President (   ) that he has successfully improved the country's economy.

4. Global warming is a/an (   ) phenomenon.

5. Breakfast in our family includes various kinds of (   ) food.

6. The Japanese (　　　　　　) is said to be rich in vegetables and fish.

7. The suspect finally (　　　　　　) that he committed the crime.

8. We have (　　　　　　) what we originally planned to do

9. My husband and I have to (　　　　　　) our children and pets.

10. What (　　　　　　) you from coming on time?

✍ Comprehension

Underline the words in each sentence that don't match the content of the article and correct them.

1. Each year more than 11 million early deaths will take place.

   ⇒ (　　　　　　　　　　　　　　　　　　　　　　　　　　　)

2. The life we live and how we understand it determine the health of people and the planet, and we are currently getting this seriously wrong.

   ⇒ (　　　　　　　　　　　　　　　　　　　　　　　　　　　)

3. So, what do you change to make a working health diet?

   ⇒ (　　　　　　　　　　　　　　　　　　　　　　　　　　　)

4. Saving enough money for vegetables would need big changes in other areas.

   ⇒ (　　　　　　　　　　　　　　　　　　　　　　　　　　　)

5. For Scientists doing nothing is maybe a good choice.

   ⇒ (　　　　　　　　　　　　　　　　　　　　　　　　　　　)

ⓘ Coffee Break

How does our diet impact our environment?

Americans demand cheap food, so American agricultural policy for the past 30 years has focused on providing large amounts of inexpensive calories. Two of the cheapest sources of calories are corn and soy.

Corn and soy are prized because they can be efficiently grown on vast farms. But growing just one crop consistently (a monoculture) depletes the soil and forces farmers to use greater amounts of pesticides and fertilizers.

The effects of pesticides and fertilizers on natural wildlife and a water supply are well-documented. Currently, the "dead zone" in the Gulf of Mexico, where no fish or other animals can live, has grown to 8,543 square miles.

Source: https://www.takingcharge.csh.umn.edu/explore-healing-practices/
food-medicine/how-are-food-and-environ

🗣 Words & Phrases

deplete: を枯渇させる、消耗させる
pesticide: 殺虫剤
fertilizer: （化学）肥料
well-documented: 文書で十分に裏付けられた
the Gulf of Mexico: メキシコ湾

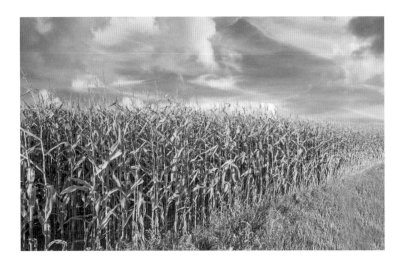

Unit 14

Edible Insects

⌘Pre-reading⌘

虫を食べるという考えは多くの人には受け入れ難いと思われます。日本でも食虫は一般的ではないですが、昔から地域によっては蜂の子やイナゴなどは食べられています。従来の食糧が、増え続ける地球の人口を支えきれない可能性のある近未来のために、たんぱく質、ミネラル、良質脂肪の宝庫であるこの小さな生き物を育て販売している施設があります。

⌘Reading⌘

It may sound sickening to some of you, but many people can and do eat insects.

Edible insects are a great source of high quality protein and minerals known to be important to good health, like calcium and iron. Insect larvae, or young, offer all that, as well as high quality fat, which is good for brain development.

Insects are food in many parts of the world, but not in the United States. In the U.S., concerns about and even fear of the creatures mean serving insects as meals is extremely rare.

But that is starting to change.

Wendy Lu McGill is opening a shipping container in a community just outside Denver, Colorado. She steps into a little room that is lined with small white boxes. Machines keep the room's temperature around 26 degrees Celsius. The relative humidity, or level of wetness in the air, is 80 percent. The conditions are just right for the extremely small creatures McGill is raising: mealworms.

"Rocky Mountain Micro Ranch is Colorado's first and only edible insect farm. We raise crickets and mealworms to sell to restaurants and food manufacturers."

The United Nations Food and Agricultural Organization has said that the world's demand for protein from beef and even chicken is unsustainable. Protein from bugs is one possible solution.

McGill grows nearly 275 kilograms of insects every month. She feeds them crushed, wet grain. A carrot supplies their water needs. Each mealworm is about half the size of the smallest finger on a human hand. Thousands of the insects bend and move in each shallow container.

"I want to be part of trying to figure out how to feed ourselves better as we have less land and water and a hotter planet and more people to feed."

Visiting McGill's Micro Ranch today are Terry Koelling and his grand-children. Andrew is almost five years old and Zora is nearly three. Like most Americans, they have never ever eaten a bug. They do not seem to want to try one now, either. 30

"I don't think they are very appealing, as far as something you put in your mouth. And you see them around dead things, and it just doesn't ap-peal to me to eat something that seems to be so wild." 35

Another visitor to the insect farm already likes the idea of using bugs as food.

"I'm Amy Franklin and I'm founder of a non-profit called Farms for Orphans. And what we do is farm bugs for food because in other countries where we work, they are a really, really popular food." 40

Franklin works in the Democratic Republic of Congo. In its markets, people sell live wild-caught crickets and African Palm weevil larvae to eat. These wild insects are only plentiful seasonally.

Franklin says some Congolese orphanages grow African Palm weevil larvae year round in shipping containers. 45

"Most of the orphanages don't own any land. There really is no oppor-tunity for them to grow a garden or to raise chickens. Insects are a protein source that they can grow in a very small space."

🐝 Words & Phrases ───────────────────────────

[l. 4]   **larvae:** larva の複数形、幼虫

[l. 16] **mealworm:** ゴミムシダマシ科の昆虫の幼虫の総称

[l. 17] **Rocky Mountain Micro Ranch:** コロラド州の最初で唯一の食用虫を育てている農場

[l. 20] **The United Nations Food and Agricultural Organization:** 国際連合食糧農業機関

[l. 41] **Democratic Republic of Congo:** コンゴ民主共和国

[l. 42] **African Palm weevil:** アフリカヤシゾウムシ

☑Vocabulary Check

Match each word in the box with the most appropriate definition shown below.

Words	Definitions	Words	Definitions
sickening		bug	
ship		appeal	
relative		found	
raise		orphan	
unsustainable		plentiful	

Definitions:

a. a child whose parents are dead or not present
b. send, transport
c. a small insect
d. a characteristic measured in comparison to something else
e. bring up or grow
f. establish or originate
g. not able to be maintained
h. existing in great quantities
i. disgusting
j. attract

♀ Vocabulary Practice

Complete the following sentences with the words shown in the box. Change the grammatical form if necessary.

1. I was born and (   ) in a small city near Osaka.

2. The discount price for the new TV was very (   ) to my mom and dad.

3. Oliver Twist, a hero of Charles Dickens' famous novel, lives in a/an (   ).

4. The current rate of population growth will be (   ) in the near future.

5. Winter in this country is (   ) mild.

6. The (   ) day of the university is in May.

7. The harvest of apples in this area is (   ).

8. The (   ) smell of the spilt chemicals from the factory chased all the local people away.

9. The product will be (   ) immediately after the payment has been secured.

10. Some people are allergic to certain kinds of (   ).

✍ Comprehension

Read the following sentences on the content of the article and choose the best answer.

1. What can insects provide as a source of food for human beings?

    a. an unusual snack for surprising your friends
    b. more energy than vegetables and grains
    c. high quality protein and minerals
    d. chances to overcome fears and feelings of disgust

2. In the United States, how common is it for people to serve insects as a meal?

    a. It is a daily part of breakfast for Americans.
    b. It is normal for children because they eat them in school lunches.
    c. It has become more popular in recent years.
    d. It is extremely rare and people are afraid of them.

3. What four problems in the future does Wendy Lu McGill say will make it difficult for us to feed ourselves like we do now? (Choose two answers)

    a. We will have less land and water.
    b. We will have less time to work and more debt.
    c. We will have more poor people and fewer farms.
    d. We will have a hotter planet and more people to feed.

4. Why does Amy Franklin want orphans to raise insects for people to eat?

    a. It will help people to overcome their fears.
    b. Many insects are edible and a good source of sugar.
    c. Selling insects as food is a good way to make money.
    d. Insects are more delicious than beef and chicken.

5. If people are poor or don't have land to do farming, where can they raise insects for food?

    a. They can raise insects in trees near where they live.

    b. They can raise insects in old fruit that they can get for free.

    c. They can raise insects in pools where the water doesn't move.

    d. They can raise insects in a shipping container instead of using land.

ⓘ Coffee Break

Eating Bugs in Japan

You may think this is rare, but Japan has bug eating traditions that are similar to other Asian countries. The oldest records of Japanese entomophagy (bug eating) are from the Edo period. Insects were eaten mostly in farming villages, but during World War II, the practice spread all over Japan. Food was scarce and bugs were readily available. But in the postwar period, more food options became available and the insect population decreased due to pesticide use, so bug eating became less common. Very few people in Japan were eating bugs by choice…until recently. Today, there is a movement led by gourmet chefs, activists, authors, and food experts who are promoting insects as a delicious food of the future.

Source: https://www.tofugu.com/japan/eating-bugs/:

📖 Words & Phrases ─────────────────────────

entomophagy: 食虫習慣
pesticide: 殺虫剤、殺菌剤、除草剤

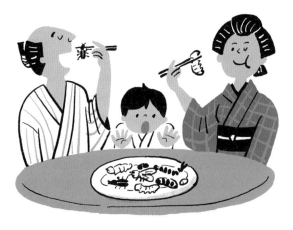

Unit 15

Medical Comics

⌘Pre-reading⌘

益々多くのコミックが病院の検査室や治療室に登場しています。特に年少の子供達がしり込みする検査や治療も、彼らがコミックを読むことにより、検査や薬の働きが面白くわかりやすくなるので怖がらなくなるためです。大学病院では医学生に、病気に立ち向かう患者を理解する上で重要な様々なテーマを教える為にもコミックを使っています。

⌘Reading⌘

A growing number of comics and graphic novels are finding their way into medical exam rooms. Experts say that especially for young patients, comics can be a great tool to explain what can be a scary medical process in an easy and entertaining manner. Comics also play a role for adults and emergency room doctors. The increasing and varied use of graphic arts 5 was the focus of a recent Comics and Medicine conference at Johns Hopkins Medical Campus in Maryland.

Medications are the heroes and allergens become villains in the Iggy and The Inhalers series. Alex Thomas, a pediatric allergist at the University of Wisconsin, uses this video and other comics he created for his asthma 10 patients with his partner Gary Ashwal, a health communications specialist.

"What we are trying to do is to insert scientific information into those metaphors so that kids are excited to be learning about super heroes and learning about super villains, and their strength and their weakness without kind of realizing they are actually learning about asthma pathology, 15 asthma triggers and the correct use of medications, and the mechanisms of action," said Thomas.

There are no significant statistics yet on the effectiveness of comics as an educational tool, but, Thomas says, his tests show promising results.

"For example, one of the questions was how does a 'Bronchodilator' 20 work as a type of asthma medication. Before the comic book, 18 percent kids got it right. After the comic book, 68 percent kids got it right," he said.

The use of comics is not limited to children. Brian Kloss is an emergency medicine physician at SUNY Upstate Medical University in New York. He recently published "Toxicology in a Box." It contains 150 flash- 25 cards he uses to teach medical students to recognize and treat drug overdoses and poisonings.

The Comics and Medicine conference included sessions where doctors learned about using comics in their practices and workshops on how to draw them. 30

"I use them [comics] a lot in my teaching with medical students as a way of helping explore various themes that I think are really important for doctors understanding the patient's experience of illness and how to understand complicated stories," explained Michael Green, a doctor of Internal Medicine at the Penn State College of Medicine. 35

There are also a growing number of cartoon style memoirs on illness, including the New York Times bestseller, "Marbles." Ellen Forney, who chronicled her struggle with bipolar disorder, was a keynote speaker at the conference.

"I think that comics are a medium that is really, really powerful for telling 40 personal stories," said Forney.

Comics are still a small part of the healing arts, but doctors who use them say they play an increasingly important role.

📖 Words & Phrases

[l. 6] **Comics and Medicine conference at John Hopkins Medical Campus:** ジョンズ・ホプキンズ大学医学部とペンシルベニア州立大学医学部の共同開催による『コミックと医学』をテーマにした会議
[l. 8] **allergen:** アレルゲン、アレルギー起因物質
[l. 8] **Iggy and The Inhalers:** 子供のために喘息をわかりやすく説明した漫画雑誌
[l. 9] **allergist:** アレルギー専門医
[l. 11] **health communication:** 医療コミュニケーション学。医療、公衆衛生の分野において医学研究の成果を、医療従事者のみでなく医療消費者をも含めた効率的な情報共有をめざす考え方
[l. 20] **bronchodilator:** 気管支拡張剤
[l. 24] **SUNY Upstate Medical University:** SUNYアップステート・メディカル大学
[l. 25] **toxicology:** 毒物学
[l. 34] **internal medicine:** 内科医学
[l. 35] **Penn State College of Medicine:** ペンステイト医科大学（ペンシルベニア州立大学医学部）
[l. 37] **Marbles:** 漫画家エレン・フォニー（1968～）のベストセラー自伝漫画（2012年）
[l. 38] **bipolar disorder:** 双極性障害、躁鬱病

☑Vocabulary Check

Match each word in the box with the most appropriate definition shown below.

Words	Definitions	Words	Definitions
villain		significant	
pediatric		promising	
insert		memoir	
metaphor		chronicle	
pathology		medium	

Definitions:

a. seems likely to be successful

b. an imaginative way of describing something by referring to something else

c. a biography written from personal knowledge

d. a person capable of doing harm or evil

e. the branch of medicine dealing with children and their diseases

f. the study of the way diseases and illnesses develop

g. place or push into something else

h. something which is used to deliver something else

i. important, large enough

j. an account or record of a series of events

♀ Vocabulary Practice

Complete the following sentences with the words shown in the box. Change the grammatical form if necessary.

1. English is used as the (   ) of conferences worldwide.

2. The virus affected a/an (   ) amount of people.

3. The (   ) of Narnia is a very exciting series of fantasy novels by C.S. Lewis.

4. That American actor is so good at playing the role of a/an (   ).

5. When my mother got older, she decided to write a/an (   ) of her life.

6. This small pin should be (   ) into a mobile phone to remove the SIM card.

7. He is one of the most (   ) students. He will surely be successful.

8. The (   ) department of the hospital is always busy with sick children.

9. Patients have to wait until scientists fully understand the (   ) of lung cancer.

10. Using a/an (   ) is an effective way of delivering a speech.

✎ Comprehension

Choose the correct phrase to complete the sentence in line with the article.

1. The increasing and varied use of graphic arts (   ) a recent Comics and Medicine conference.
- **a.** became popular at
- **b.** has been explored in
- **c.** was examined at
- **d.** might have influenced

2. There are no significant statistics yet (   ) comics as an educational tool.
- **a.** being used in
- **b.** about the benefits of
- **c.** published and studied about
- **d.** available regarding

3. "Toxicology in a Box" contains 150 flashcards used to teach medical students (   ) drug overdoses and poisonings.
- **a.** about the dangers of
- **b.** in order to keep them safe from
- **c.** who are interested in
- **d.** to identify and deal with

4. The Comics and Medicine conference included sessions (   )
   using comics in their practices and workshops on how to draw them.

      a. in which caregivers are taught about

      b. where artists experience

      c. designed for people who are

      d. researching writers with success in

5. Ellen Forney thinks that comics are a (   ) powerful for telling
   personal stories.

      a. fun art form and can be

      b. popular thing but not so

      c. profitable tool because they are

      d. method which is very

ⓘ Coffee Break

Coronavirus Symptoms

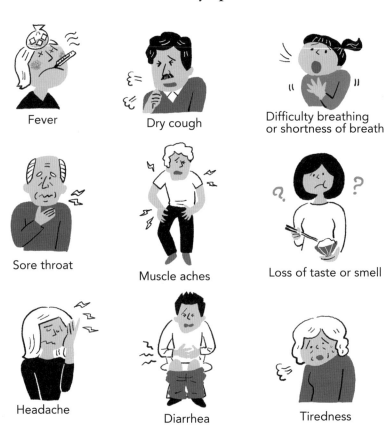

Fever

Dry cough

Difficulty breathing
or shortness of breath

Sore throat

Muscle aches

Loss of taste or smell

Headache

Diarrhea

Tiredness

Appendix I

① List of Common Diseases in English
（代表的な疾患名称リスト）

頭部の病気　brain diseases
髄膜炎　meningitis
脳炎　encephalitis : inflammation of the brain
脳腫瘍　cerebral tumor
髄膜腫　meningioma
ウィルス性髄膜炎　viral meningitis
神経膠芽細胞腫　glioblastoma
脳梗塞　cerebral (brain)infarction
脳出血　cerebral (brain) hemorrhage

胸部の病気　chest diseases
肺炎　pneumonia
ウィルス性肺炎　viral pneumonia
肺がん　lung cancer
肺血栓塞栓症(エコノミークラス症候群)　economy class syndrome
気胸　pneumothorax
大動脈解離　aortic dissection
心筋梗塞　myocardial infarction
狭心症　angina
乳癌　breast cancer
食道癌　esophageal cancer

腹部の病気　abdominal diseases
腸炎　inflammation of the intestines
ウィルス性腸炎　viral enteritis
虫垂炎　appendicitis
胃潰瘍　an ulcer of the stomach, a gastric ulcer
胆嚢炎　inflammation of the gallbladder, cholecystitis
膵炎　pancreatitis
肝炎　hepatitis
膀胱炎　inflammation of the bladder
尿路結石　a urinary calculus
子宮筋腫　a myoma of the uterus

胃炎　gastritis

逆流性食道炎　reflux esophagitis

胃癌　gastric cancer, stomach cancer

胆嚢癌　gallbladder cancer

肝癌　liver cancer

膵臓がん　pancreatic cancer

腎癌　kidney cancer, renal cancer

膀胱癌　bladder cancer

子宮癌　uterine cancer, cancer of the uterus (womb)

卵巣癌　ovarian cancer

腸閉塞　ileus, intestinal obstruction

感覚器（官）の病気　sensory organ diseases

白内障　cataract

緑内障　glaucoma

近視　myopia

網膜剥離　amotio retinae

麦粒腫　sty

難聴　hypoacusis (hearing loss)

メニエール病　Meniere's disease

内耳炎　inner-ear inflammation (infection)

中耳炎　middle-ear inflammation (infection)

副鼻腔炎　(paranasal) sinusitis

皮膚の病気　skin diseases

アトピー性皮膚炎　Atopic dermatitis

悪性黒色腫　malignant melanoma

粉瘤　atheroma

整形外科疾患　plastic surgery disorders

骨折　fracture

変形性関節症　osteoarthritis

血液内科疾患　hematology diseases

白血病　leukemia

リンパ腫　lymphoma

代謝内科系の病気　metabolic diseases
　　　糖尿病　diabetes
　　　バセドウ病　Basedow disease, Graves' disease

精神科疾患　psychiatric disorders
　　　うつ病　depression
　　　統合失調症　schizophrenia
　　　躁鬱病　manic depression

② Common Names of Diagnosis and Treatment Departments in Japanese Hospitals
（日本の病院によく見られる診療科 [1]）

内科　Internal Medicine
　　　呼吸器内科　Respiratory Medicine
　　　循環器内科　Cardiovascular Medicine
　　　消化器内科　Gastrointestinal Medicine
　　　神経内科　Neurology
　　　代謝内科　Internal Medicine

外科　Surgery
　　　呼吸器外科　Respiratory Surgery
　　　消化器外科　Digestive Surgery
　　　心臓血管外科　Cardiovascular Surgery
　　　脳外科　Brain Surgery

小児科　Pediatrics
産婦人科　Obstetrics and Gynecology
皮膚科　Dermatology
整形外科(形成外科)　Formation Surgery
耳鼻科　Otolaryngology
精神科　Psychiatry
放射線科　Radiology

1　ここに紹介する英語表記は日本の総合病院によく見る診療科の日本語名称に基づいています。

麻酔科　**Anesthesiology**
泌尿器科　**Urology**

③ **Medical and Surgical Services in an American Hospital**[2]
（アメリカの病院によく見る医療サービス）

Allergy, Immunology and Pulmonology
　アレルギー、免疫及び肺臓
Alzheimer's Disease
　アルツハイマー型認知症
Anesthesiology
　麻酔
Arteriovenous Malformations (AVM)
　動静脈奇形 (A VM)
Autism and the Developing Brain
　自閉症・脳の発達
Blood Disorders (Hematology)
　血液疾患（血液学）
Borderline Personality Disorder Resource Center
　境界性パーソナリティー障害情報センター
Brain and Spine Trauma
　脳脊髄外傷
Brain and Spine Tumors
　脳脊髄腫瘍
Breast Centers
　乳腺センター
Burn Treatment
　熱傷処置
Cancer Services
　がんに関する医療サービス
Cancer Screening and Awareness
　がん検診・がんに対する意識学習

2　アメリカの病院の診療科は、より詳細に記載されている場合が多いです。一例として、ここでは New York Presbyterian Hospital（ニューヨークプレスビテリアン病院）のケースを紹介します。提供できる医療サービスはアルファベット順にリストアップされています。
　https://www.nyp.org/clinical-services

Cardiothoracic Surgery
胸部心臓外科

Carotid Stenosis
頸動脈狭窄症

Cerebral Aneurysm
脳動脈瘤

Cerebrovascular Disease
脳血管疾患

Children's Health (Pediatrics)
子供の健康(小児科)

Colon and Rectal Surgery
結腸・直腸手術

Craniofacial Surgery
頭蓋顔面外科

Dental, Oral and Maxillofacial Surgery
歯、口腔及び顎顔外科

Dermatology
皮膚科

Diabetes and Endocrinology
糖尿・内分泌科

Digestive Diseases
消化器系疾患

Ear, Nose, and Throat (Otolaryngology – Head & Neck Surgery)
耳・鼻・喉(耳鼻咽喉科-頭&首外科)

ECMO (Extracorporeal membrane oxygenation)
ECMO（体外式膜型人工肺）

Endocrine Surgery
内分泌外科

Epilepsy
てんかん

General Gynecology
一般婦人科

General Surgery
一般外科

Geriatrics
高齢者医療

Hand Surgery
手の手術

Head and Neck Surgery
　頭・首の手術

Heart Services
　心臓に関する医療サービス

Infectious Diseases/International Medicine
　感染病/国際医療

Integrative Health and Wellbeing Program
　総合医療福祉プログラム

Internal Medicine
　内科

Men's Health
　メンズヘルス(男性特有の疾患の関する医療)

Multiple Sclerosis
　多発性硬化症(MS)

Nephrology (Kidney Disease)
　腎臓病

Neurocritical Care
　神経集中治療

Neurological Autoimmune Disorders
　神経系自己免疫疾患

Neuromuscular Disorders
　神経筋疾患

Nutrition
　栄養

Ophthalmology (Eye)
　眼科

Ophthalmological Surgery
　眼科手術

Orthopedic Services
　整形外科に関する医療サービス

Pain Medicine
　疼痛医療

Palliative Care for Adults
　成人向け緩和ケア

Parkinsons Disease and Movement Disorders
　パーキンソン病及び運動障害

Pathology
　病理診断

Pediatric Services
小児科に関する医療サービス

Pediatric Surgery
小児外科

Plastic Surgery
形成外科

Pregnancy & Maternity Care
妊娠&出産ケア

Preventive Medicine and Nutrition
予防医療及び栄養

Psychiatry and Mental Health
精神科及びメンタルヘルス

Pulmonary Hypertension
肺高血圧症

Rehabilitation Medicine
リハビリテーション医療

Radiation Oncology
放射線腫瘍

Radiology
放射線治療

Rheumatology
リュウマチ

Sleep Disorders
睡眠障害

Spine Disorders
脊椎疾患

Stroke
脳卒中

Thoracic Surgery
胸部手術

Transplant Services
臓器移植に関する医療サービス

Trauma Care
外傷治療

Urology
泌尿器科

Weight Loss Surgery
減量手術

Women's Health
   ウーマンズヘルス(女性特有の疾患の関する医療)
Youth Anxiety
   青年期特有の不安障害

Appendix II

Medical Terminology (Root, Prefix and Suffix)

　医学用語には、複雑で馴染みにくい単語が多く存在しますが、その単語を、意味の中枢となる部分と文法的機能を表す部分にそれぞれ分割して、語幹（root/stem）と接辞（affix）を知ることで、知らない単語でも、ある程度その意味を推測することが可能な場合があります。以下に医学用語に関する基本的な語幹と接辞（接頭辞/prefix &接尾辞/suffix）を紹介します。

　ここでは、ある単語の中で基盤となる意味を持つ最小単位のことを語幹（root）と呼び、語幹だけで成立している単語もあれば、語幹に接辞がくっついて成立している単語もあります。医学用語の語幹は様々な言語（ギリシア語、ラテン語、ドイツ語やアラビア語など）に由来しています。接頭辞（prefix）は、語幹の前に現れ、後続する語幹の意味範囲を限定したり、位置関係を示したりします。接尾辞（suffix）は、語幹の後ろに現れます。医学用語の接尾辞は、品詞の派生機能だけでなく、疾患状況、手術方法や診断状況などを表すものもあります。

Roots Used in Medical Terms	Meanings (Japanese)	Examples (Japanese)
abdomin(o)-	abdomen（腹部）	abdominoscopy（腹腔鏡検査）
acou-	hearing（聴覚）	acoustics（音響学）
aden-	gland（分泌線）	adenocarcinoma（腺がん）
andr(o)-	male	androsterone（男性ホルモン）
arthr(o)-	joint（関節）	arthritis（関節炎）
bi(o)-	life	biocide（殺生物剤）
bronchi-	bronchi（気管支）	bronchitis（気管支炎）
carcin(o)-	cancer	carcinogen（発がん物質）
cardi(o)-	heart	cardiopathy（心臓病）
cephal(o)-	head	cephalalgia（頭痛）
chem(o)-	chemical	chemotherapy（化学療法）
col(i)(o)-	colon（結腸）	colitis（大腸炎）
derm-	skin	dermatitis（皮膚炎）
encephal(o)-	brain	encephaloma（脳腫瘍）
febri-	fever	febrile（熱のある）〈adj.〉
gastoro-	stomach	gastritis（胃炎）
geront(o)-	aging	gerontology（老年病学）
gloss(o)(a)-	tongue	glossitis（舌炎）
h(a)eme(a)(o)-	blood	hematology（血液学）

hepat(o)-	liver	hepatitis （肝炎）
hydro-	water	dehydrate （脱水状態になる・する）〈vi, vt〉※
leuk(o)-	white	leukemia （白血病）
mamm(o)-	breast	mammography （マンモグラフィー、乳房X線）
mast(o)-	breast	mastectomy （乳腺切除）
melan(o)-	black	melanoma （悪性黒色腫、メラノーマ）
myc(o)-	fungus （菌類）	mycosis （真菌症）
nas(o)-	nose	nasal （鼻の）〈adj.〉
nephr(o)-	kidney	nephritis （腎炎）
neur(o)-	nerve	neurologist （神経学者）
ocul(o)-	eye	intraocular （眼球内の）〈adj.〉
ophthalm(o)-	eye	ophthalmoplegia （眼筋麻痺）
oste(o)-	bone	osteitis （骨炎）
p(a)ed(o)-	child	pediatrics （小児科）
path(o)-	disease	pathogen （病原体）
pharmac(o)-	drugs	pharmaceutical （薬剤の、薬剤）〈adj. n.〉
pneum(o)-	lung	pneumonia （肺炎）
pod(o)-	foot	podiatry （足病学、足治療）
psych(o)-	mind	psychiatrist （精神科医）
ren(o)-	kidney	renography （レノグラフィー、腎撮影）
sten(o)-	narrow （狭い）	stenosis （狭窄症）
therm(o)-	heat	thermography （サーモグラフィー）
ven(i)(o)-	vein （静脈）	intravenous injection （IV, 静脈注射、点滴）

※　vi: 自動詞、vt: 他動詞、n.: 名詞、adj.: 形容詞を示す。尚、特記なしの場合は、医学用語として
　　主に名詞で使用される。

Prefixes Used in Medical Terms	Meanings (Japanese)	Examples (Japanese)
a/an-	without, lack of	anuria（無尿症）
ab-	away from	abnormal（異常の）〈adj.〉
ambi-	both sides	ambidextrous（両手利きの、器用な）〈adj.〉
anti-	against	antibiotic（抗生物質、抗生物質の）〈n. /adj.〉
auto-	self	autograft（自家移植する、自家移植）〈vt. /adj.〉
bi-	both, two	bilateral（両側に発生する、左右対称の）〈adj.〉
con-	with, together	congenital（先天性の、本来備わっている）〈adj.〉
de-	without	depigmentation（脱色）cf. pigment: 色素
diplo-	double	diplopia（複視）cf. -opia: 視覚異常
dys-	difficult, painful	dyspnea（呼吸困難）
endo-	within, inside	endoscope（内視鏡）
epi-	above	epigastric（上腹部の）〈adj.〉
eu-	normal	euthyroid（甲状腺機能正常の）〈adj.〉
ex-	outward（外側の）	exostosis（外骨腫症）
extra-	outside of	extrapleural（胸膜外の）〈adj.〉
hemi-	half	hemiplegia（片麻痺）
hetero-	different	heterograft（異種移植する、異種移植）〈n. vt.〉
homo-	same	homoplasty（同種移植術）
hyper-	excessive（過度の）	hyperactive（異常に活発な）
hypo-	deficient（不足した）	hypotension（低血圧症）=low blood pressure
in-	not, inward	infertility（不妊症）
inter-	between	intervertebral（椎間の）〈adj.〉
intra-	within	intravenous（静脈内の）〈adj.〉
juxta-	near	juxta-articular（関節近接の）〈adj.〉
macro-	large	macroglossia（巨大舌）
mal-	bad, abnormal	malnutrition（栄養失調）
micro-	small	microorganism（微生物）
mono-	one	monochromatic（全視覚異常の、単一色しか見えない）〈adj.〉
morph(o)-	shape	morphology（≪生物≫形態学、≪言語≫形態論）
multi-	many	multigravida（経妊婦、妊娠経験のある女性）
neo-	new	neonatal（新生児の）〈adj.〉
nulli-	none	nullipara（未産婦）
pan-	all	panacea（万能薬）
par(a)-	beside, abnormal	parasite（寄生生物）
per-	through	percutaneous（経皮の）〈adj.〉 cf. cutaneous: 皮膚の

pico-	one-trillionth （1兆分の1）	picornavirus（ピコルナウイルス、極めて小さいRNA ウイルス）
poly-	many, much	polyuria（多尿症）
post-	after	postpartum（分娩後の）〈adj.〉
pre-	before	precancer（前がん状態）
pseudo-	false	pseudocyesis（想像妊娠、偽妊娠）
re-	again	reinfection（再感染）
retr(o)-	backward	retrograde（退化する、悪化する）〈adj.〉〈vi〉
semi-	half	semicomatose（半昏睡状態の）〈adj.〉
sub-	under	subcutaneous（皮下の）〈adj.〉
supra-	above	suprarenal（副腎の）〈adj.〉
syn-	together, with	syndrome（症候群、一群の関連のあるもの）
un-	not	unconscious（意識を失った）〈adj.〉
uni-	one	unilateral（体の片側の）〈adj.〉

Suffixes Used in Medical Terms	Meanings (Japanese)	Examples (Japanese)
-algia	pain	neuralgia（神経痛）
-cyte	cell（細胞）	leucocyte（白血球）
-ectasis	dilation（拡張）	bronchiectasis（気管支拡張症）
-ectomy	surgical removal （外科的切除、摘出）	splenectomy（脾臓摘出）
-emesis	vomiting（嘔吐）	hematemesis（吐血）
-itis	inflammation（炎症）	bronchitis（気管支炎）
-ism	state of（〜の状態）	metabolism（代謝作用）
-logist	one who studies	cardiologist（心臓専門医）
-lys(i)(o)	breakdown（故障）	cytolysis（細胞崩壊）
-oma	tumor（腫瘍）	glioma（神経膠腫）
-osis	condition	fibrosis（線維症）
-pathy	disease	myopathy（筋疾患、ミオパシー）
-plasia	growth（発育）	hypoplasia（発育不全）
-plasty	surgical repair（形成）	angioplasty（血管形成）
-praxia	movement	apraxia（失行症）
-rrhea	fluid discharge （流体流出）	diarrhea（下痢）
-scope	observe	endoscope（内視鏡）
-taxis	movement	ataxia（運動失調）
-tomy	incision（切開）	caesarotomy（帝王切開）cf. C-section
-tripsy	crushing（粉砕）	lithotripsy（結石の砕石術）
-trophy	growth（増大）	hypertrophy（肥大、肥大する・させる）〈n.〉 〈vi〉 〈vt〉

Source: https://www.pharmapproach.com

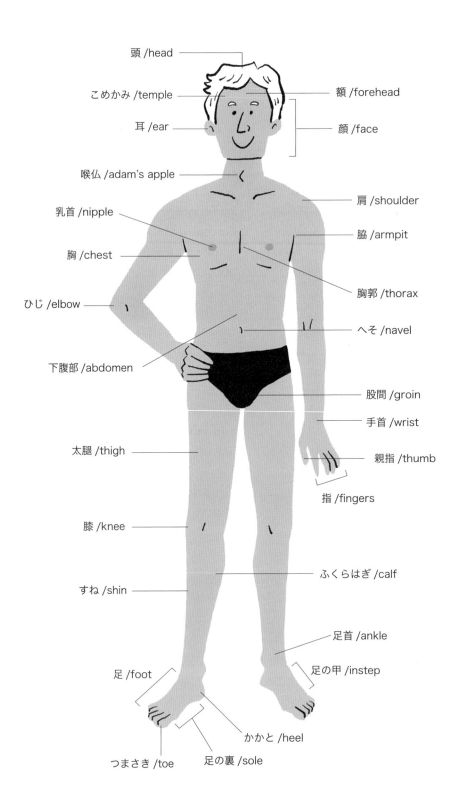

頭 /head
こめかみ /temple
耳 /ear
喉仏 /adam's apple
乳首 /nipple
胸 /chest
ひじ /elbow
下腹部 /abdomen
太腿 /thigh
膝 /knee
すね /shin
足 /foot
つまさき /toe
足の裏 /sole
かかと /heel
額 /forehead
顔 /face
肩 /shoulder
脇 /armpit
胸郭 /thorax
へそ /navel
股間 /groin
手首 /wrist
親指 /thumb
指 /fingers
ふくらはぎ /calf
足首 /ankle
足の甲 /instep

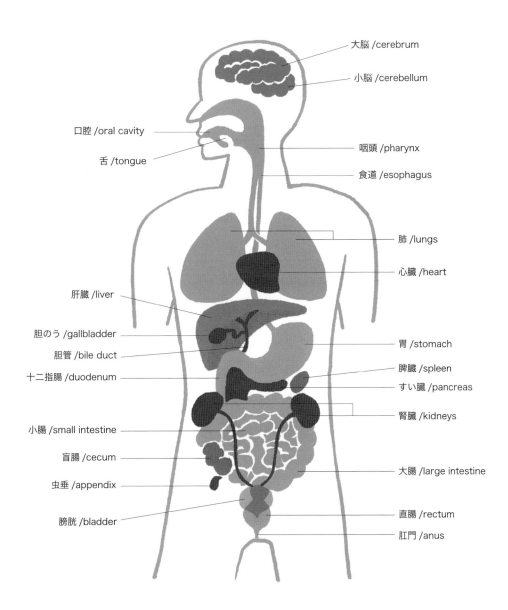

大脳 /cerebrum

小脳 /cerebellum

口腔 /oral cavity

咽頭 /pharynx

舌 /tongue

食道 /esophagus

肺 /lungs

心臓 /heart

肝臓 /liver

胆のう /gallbladder

胃 /stomach

胆管 /bile duct

脾臓 /spleen

十二指腸 /duodenum

すい臓 /pancreas

腎臓 /kidneys

小腸 /small intestine

盲腸 /cecum

大腸 /large intestine

虫垂 /appendix

膀胱 /bladder

直腸 /rectum

肛門 /anus

今求められる医療と看護

検印
省略

© 2021年1月31日　初版発行

著　者　　　　　　　　　　　吉岡みのり
　　　　　　　　　　　　Gerald R. Gordon
　　　　　　　　　　　　　　近藤　進

発行者　　　　　　　　　　　原　雅　久

発行所　　　　　　株式会社　朝 日 出 版 社
　　　　　101-0065　東京都千代田区西神田 3-3-5
　　　　　　　　電話　東京 (03) 3239-0271/72
　　　　　　　　FAX　東京 (03) 3239-0479
　　　　　e-mail　text-e@asahipress.com
　　　　　　　　振替口座　00140-2-46008
　　　組版／クロス・コンサルティング　製版／錦明印刷

乱丁・落丁はお取り替えいたします。
ISBN978-4-255-15672-9　C1082

ちょっと手ごわい、でも効果絶大!
最強のリスニング強化マガジン

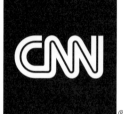 **CNN ENGLISH EXPRESS**

音声ダウンロード付き　毎月6日発売　定価(本体1,148円＋税)

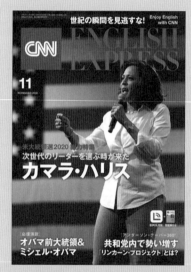

定期購読をお申し込みの方には
本誌1号分無料ほか、特典多数。
詳しくは下記ホームページへ。

英語が楽しく続けられる!

重大事件から日常のおもしろネタ、
スターや著名人のインタビューなど、
CNNの多彩なニュースを
生の音声とともにお届けします。
3段階ステップアップ方式で
初めて学習する方も安心。
どなたでも楽しく続けられて
実践的な英語力が身につきます。

資格試験の強い味方!

ニュース英語に慣れれば、TOEIC ®テストや英検の
リスニング問題も楽に聞き取れるようになります。

CNN ENGLISH EXPRESS ホームページ

英語学習に役立つコンテンツが満載!

[本誌のホームページ] https://ee.asahipress.com/
[編集部のTwitter] https://twitter.com/asahipress_ee

朝日出版社 〒101-0065 東京都千代田区西神田 3-3-5　TEL 03-3263-3321

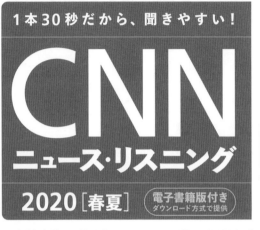
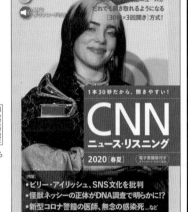

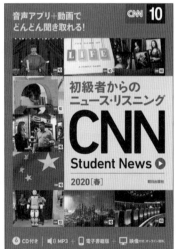

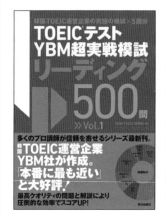
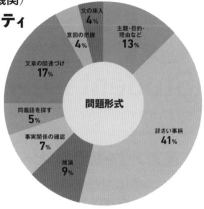

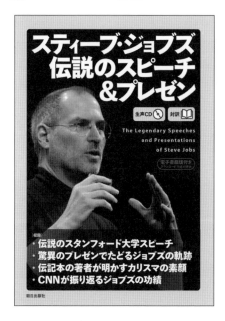